Readings in

DYSLEXIA

Special Learning Corporation
42 Boston Post Rd. Guilford, Connecticut 06437

SPECIAL LEARNING CORPORATION

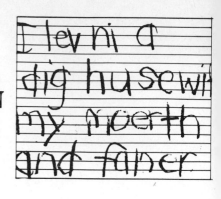

Publisher's Message:

The Special Education Series is the first comprehensive series designed for special education courses of study. It is also the first series to offer such a wide variety of high quality books. In addition, the series will be expanded and up-dated each year. No other publications in the area of special education can equal this. We stress high quality content, a superb advisory and consulting group, and special features that help in understanding the course of study. In addition we believe we must also publish in very small enrollment areas in order to establish the credibility and strength of our series. We realize the enrollments in courses of study such as Autism, Visually Handicapped Education, or Diagnosis and Placement are not large. Nevertheless, we believe there is a need for course books in these areas and books that are kept up-to-date on an annual basis! Special Learning Corporation's goal is to publish the highest quality materials for the college and university courses of study. With your comments and support we will continue to do this.

John P. Quirk

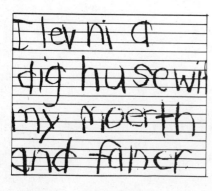

First Edition
1 2 3 4 5

ISBN No.   0-89568-014-9

Manufactured by the Redson Rice Corporation, Chicago, Illinois

SPECIAL EDUCATION SERIES

- ● Autism
- • ● Behavior Modification
-   Biological Bases of Learning Disabilities
-   Brain Impairments
-   Career and Vocational Education
-   Child Abuse
-   Child Development
-   Child Psychology
-   Cognitive and Communication Skills
-   Creative Arts
-   **Curriculum and Materials**
- • ● Deaf Education
-   Developmental Disabilities
- • ● Diagnosis and Placement
-   Down's Syndrome
- ● Dyslexia
-   Early Learning
-   Educational Technology
- • ● Emotional and Behavioral Disorders
-   Exceptional Parents

- • ● Gifted Education
-   Hyperactivity
- • ● Learning Disabilities
-   Learning Theory
- ● Mainstreaming
- • ● Mental Retardation
-   Multiple Handicapped Education
-   Occupational Therapy
- • ● Physically Handicapped Education
-   **Pre-School and Day Care Education**
- • ● Psychology of Exceptional Children
-   Reading Skill Development
-   Research and Development
-   Severe Mental Retardation
-   Slow Learner Education
-   Social Learning
- • ● Special Education
- • ● Speech and Hearing
-   Testing and Diagnosis
- • ● Visually Handicapped Education

● Published Titles   • Major Course Areas

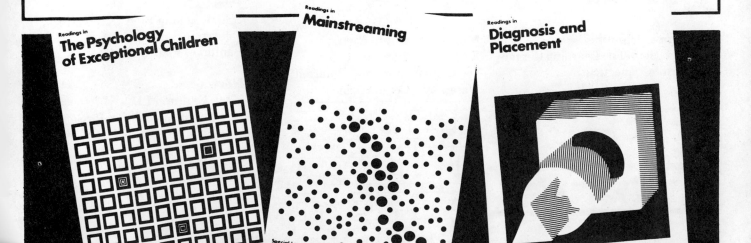

Readings in
The Psychology of Exceptional Children

Readings in
Mainstreaming

Readings in
Diagnosis and Placement

Special Learning Corporation

Special Learning Corporation

Special Learning Corporation

Dyslexia

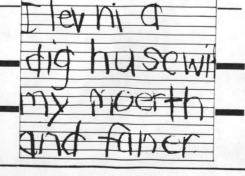

CONTENTS

1. Dyslexia – An Overview

2. Diagnosis and Assessment

Focus I   40

3. Instructional Techniques

Focus II

4. Emerging Concepts

TOPIC MATRIX

Readings in Dyslexia provides the college student in special education a comprehensive overview of the subject. The book is designed to follow a basic course of study.

COURSE OUTLINE:

Education of the Dyslexic Child

I. Diagnosis and remediation of reading disabilities

II. Special problems in reading instruction

III. Developing reading skills for the dyslexic child

IV. Measurement and evaluation of reading disorders

Readings in Dyslexia

I. Dyslexia —An Overview

II. Diagnosis and Assessment

III. Instructional Techniques

IV. Emerging Concepts

Related Special Learning Corporation Readers

I. Readings in Special Education

II. Readings in Learning Disabilities

III. Readings in Psychology of Exceptional Children

IV. Readings in Diagnosis and Placement

GLOSSARY OF TERMS

agnosia Loss of or an impairment of the ability to recognize objects or events when presented through various modalities.

alexia The loss of ability to read because of some brain damage, such as a cerebral stroke. The term also refers to the complete failure to acquire reading skills as well as to a partial or complete loss of these skills through damage.

anomia Difficulty in recalling or remembering words or the names of objects.

auditory agnosia Inability to recognize sounds or combinations of sounds without regard to their meaning.

basal reader approach A method of teaching reading in which instruction is given through the use of a series of basal readers. Sequence of skills, content, vocabulary, and activities are determined by the authors of the series. Teacher's manuals and children's activity books accompany the basal reading series.

binocular difficulties A visual impairment due to the inability of the two eyes to function together.

behavior modification A technique of changing human behavior based on the theory of operant behavior and conditioning. Careful observation of events preceding and following the behavior in question is required. The environment is manipulated to reinforce the desired responses, thereby bringing about the desired change in behavior.

bibliotherapy The use of reading, particularly the use of characters in books with whom the child identifies, for therapeutic purposes.

cerebral dominance The control of activities by the brain, with one hemisphere usually considered consistently dominant over the other. In most individuals, the left side of the brain controls language function, and the left is considered the dominant hemisphere.

cloze procedure A technique used in testing, teaching reading comprehension, and determination of readability. It involves deletion of words from the text and leaving blank spaces. Measurement is made by rating the number of blanks which can be correctly filled.

developmental imbalance A disparity in the developmental patterns of intellectual skills.

developmental reading The pattern and sequence of normal reading growth and development in a child in the learning-to-read process.

directionality Awareness of the verticle axis and awareness of the relative position of one side of the body versus the other.

discrimination The act of distinguishing differences among various stimuli.

dissociation Inability to synthesize separate and distinct elements into integrated meaningful wholes.

distractibility Forced responsiveness to extraneous stimuli.

dysfunction Disordered or impaired functioning of bodily systems.

dysgraphia Extremely poor handwriting or the inability to perform the motor movements required for handwriting. The condition is often associated with neurological dysfunction.

dyslexia A disorder of children who, despite conventional classroom experience, fail to attain the skills of reading. The term is frequently used when neurological dysfunction is suspected as the cause of the reading disability.

figure-ground distortion An inability to focus on an object itself without having the background or setting interfere with perception.

figure-ground perception The ability to attend to one aspect of the visual field while perceiving it in relation to the rest of the field.

hyperkinetic Disorganized, disruptive, and unpredictable behavior, an overreaction to stimuli.

individualized reading The method of teaching reading that utilizes the child's interest; learning is structured through the child's own reading selections, using a variety of books. The teacher acts as a consultant, aid and counselor.

laterality Involves the awareness of the two sides of one's body and the ability to identify them as left or right correctly.

learning disabilities (Based on definition provided by the National Advisory Committee on Handcapped Children, U.S. Dept. of Health, Education, and Welfare, 1968.) A learning disability refers to one or more significant deficits in essential learning processes requiring special educational techniques for its remediation. Children with learning disabilities generally demonstrate a discrepancy between expected and actual achievement in one or more areas, such as spoken, read, or written language, mathematics, and spatial orientation. The learning disability referred to is not primarily the result of sensory, motor, intellectual, or emotional handicap, or lack of opportunity to learn. Deficits are to be defined in terms of accepted diagnostic procedures in education and psychology. Essential learning processes are those currently referred to in behavioral science as perception, integration, and expression, either verbal or nonverbal. Special education techniques for remediation require educational planning based on the diagnostic procedures and findings.

memory The ability to store and retrieve upon demand previously experienced sensations and perceptions, even when the stimulus that originally evoked them is no longer present. Also referred to as "imagery" and "recall."

morpheme The smallest meaning-bearing unit in a language. which an individual receives information and thereby learns. The "modality concept" postulates that some individuals learn better through one modality than through another. For example, a child may receive data better through the visual modality than through his auditory modality.

morpheme The smallest meaning-bearing unit in a language.

ocular pursuit Eye movement that is a result of visually following a moving target.

perception The process of organizing or interpreting the raw data obtained through the senses.

perceptual constancy The ability to accurately perceive the invariant properties of objects – such as shape, position, size, etc; – in spite of the variability of the impression these objects make on the senses of the observer.

primary reading retardation The capacity to learn to read is impaired and no definite brain damage is suggested in the history or neurological examination. Further, there is no evidence of secondary reading retardation (that due to exogenous causes such as emotional disturbances or lack of opportunity). The problem seems to reflect a lack of neurological organization.

programmed reading A method of teaching reading that uses programed self-instructional and self-corrective materials.

psychoeducational diagnostician A specialist who diagnoses and evaluates a child who is having difficulty in learning. A variety of psychological and educational testing instruments are used.

psychomotor The motor effects of psychological processes and events.

readability level An indication of the difficulty of reading material in terms of the grade level at which it might be expected to be read successfully.

receptive language Language that is spoken by others and received by the individual. The receptive language skills are listening and reading.

Sensory-motor (sensorimotor) A term applied to the combination of the input of sensations and the output of motor activity. The motor activity reflects what is happening to the sensory organs such as the visual, auditory, tactual, and kinesthetic sensations.

strephosymbolia Perception of visual stimuli, especially words, in reversed or twisted order. The condition may be explained as "twisted symbols."

stimulus An external event which causes physiological change in the sense organ.

structure words (function words) Linguistic referents for words of a sentence that show the relationship between parts of the sentence as opposed to content words. Structure words include these elements of traditional grammar: prepositions, conjunctions, modal and auxiliary verbs, and articles.

syntax The grammar system of a language. The linguistic rules of word order and the function of words in a sentence.

tachistoscope A machine that exposes written material for a short period of time. Practice with such machines is designed to improve rate and span of visual perception of words.

tactile perception The ability to interpret and give meaning to sensory stimuli that are experienced through the sense of touch.

visual perception The indentification, organization, and interpretation of sensory data received by the individual through the eye.

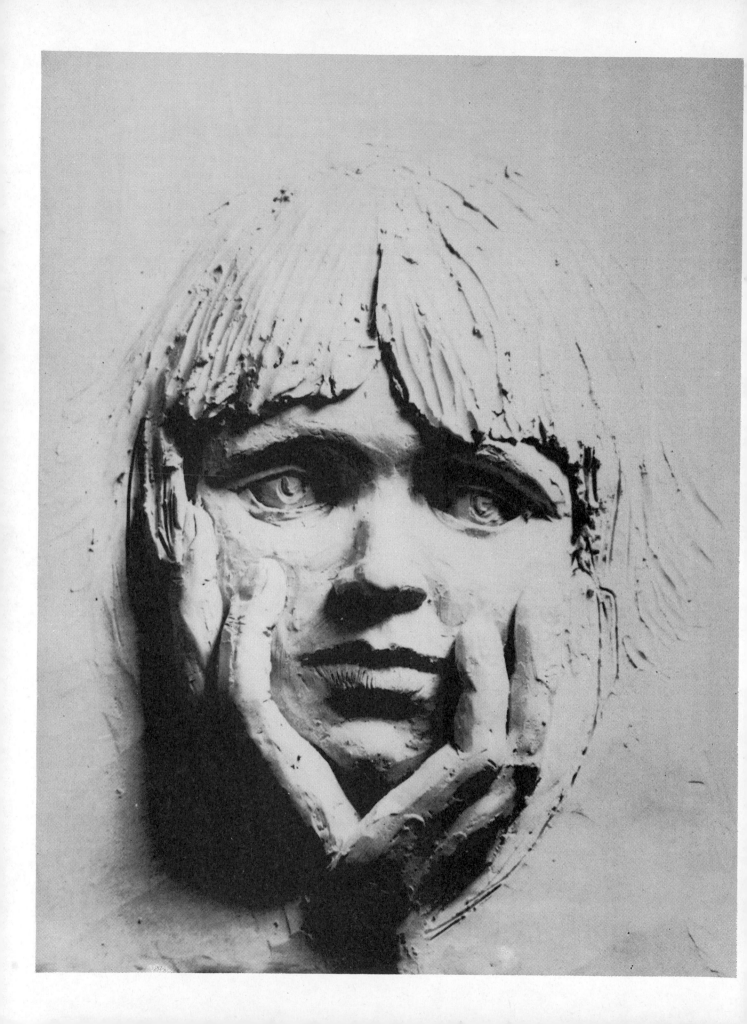

PREFACE

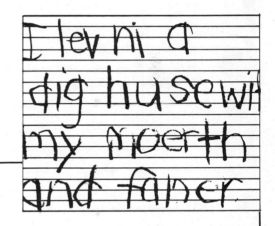

Many European educators feel there is no such thing as "dyslexia". Many American educators who have been involved in reading and learning disabilities for many years also agree. "Most of these problems work out by themselves," one leading reading teacher/author has stated. Other learning disability teachers, especially new graduates of colleges of special education, strongly disagree.

With better and improved diagnosis specific disabilities such as dyslexia are identified sooner. It is generally believed dyslexia is an impairment in the ability to read as a result of brain lesions. The dyslexic child is not different from the rest of us except his minor impairments become highly debilitating for they make it extremely difficult for him to learn to read. This effects writing and all other academic learning. This disability occurs five to six more times more often in boys than girls and is also believed to be genetic and related to left-handedness. As specialization in teacher-training occurs more and more, better teachers and better programming for remediation will be developed.

This book is designed to serve for those interested in dyslxia as a specific learning disability. Diagnosis, methods in teaching, and remediation are all discussed in great detail. Case studies are given as well. It should be pointed out the "popularity" of dyslexia demands a specific recognition of the problem – what it is – and the proper treatment and education involved with dyslexia.

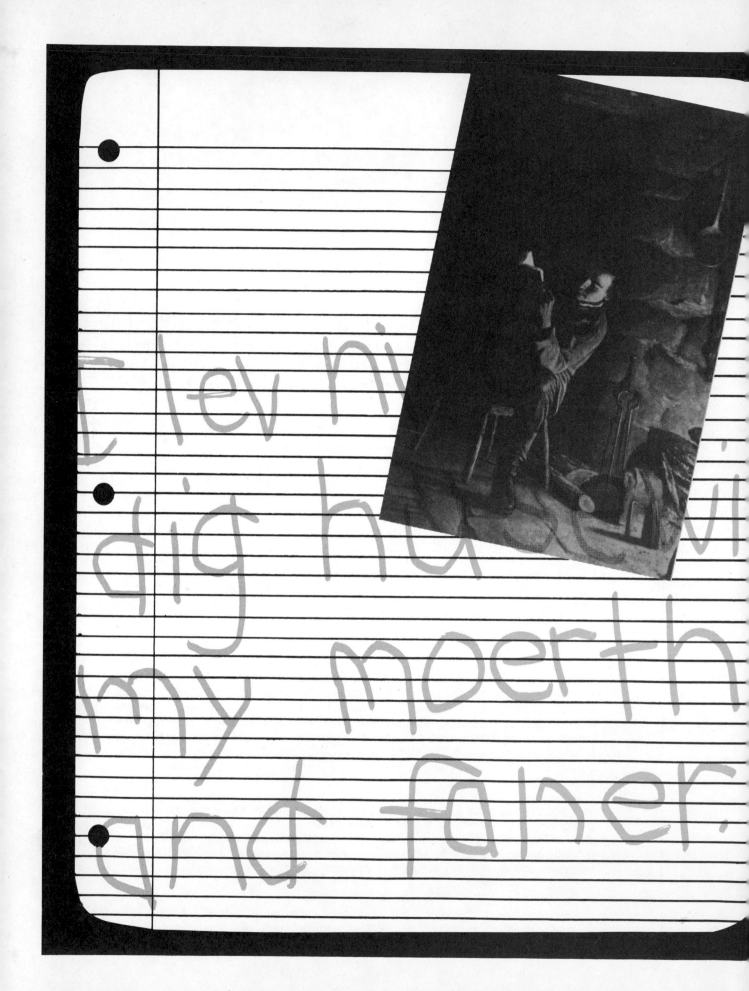

DYSLEXIA — An Overview

Historically speaking, children who experience reading disabilities have been classified according to a variety of terminology. Strephosymbolia was used in 1937 by Orton to describe the child with a "twisted" symbol difficulty. Later on, terms, such as alexia, minimal brain dysfunction and word blindness, were utilized. Most recently the term dyslexia has come into wide use to term children who experience learning disabilities in reading. Originally, the term was coined to denote children with neurological disturbances which lead to reading disturbances. Presently the word takes on many meanings, such as an indication of genetic causes for the occurrence of reading disturbance.

As far back as 1896, Morgan first reported suspected causes through various methods, techniques and materials. The medical profession made strides in research on etiology, believing that a form of brain dysfunction caused dyslexic patterns. Educators took the stand that poor and inappropriate instruction were the main factors. Today, educators attempt to identify deficient reading behaviors and design appropriate reading skills accordingly.

The process of learning to read involves many different skills and their acquisition. Generally, it is thought that the reading process is composed of recognition skills and comprehension skills. The following listing breaks down into stages the developmental process:
1. Reading readiness development
2. Conceptual stage of learning to read
3. Word recognition and reading skills
4. Structural reading
5. Refinement of reading skills

The types of problems which children may face who experience reading disabilities include inability to discriminate visually various letters or words. Auditory disturbances may produce inability to differentiate between phonemic sounds. Emphasis would then be placed on the blending of syllables and using words in meaningful context in order that remediation might begin.

Memory disturbances which affect the ability to recall information that has been learned must also be considered . . . the omission of various sounds or the order of sounds might be confusing in the sequential memory process. The most commonly recognized characteristic of the child with a reading disability is the tendency to read or write some letters and words backwards, inverted, or rotated. The inability to discriminate left from right is most often thought to be the reason for these reversals.

Taken as a whole, learning disabilities in reading include these factors – major word recognition, comprehension skill deficiency levels, word analysis which can be remediated through informal diagnostic techniques, which might include informal reading inventory, standardized reading testing and the most current popular reading methods.

Although educators, reading specialists and psychologists might generally adopt different views of dyslexia and what it is, the Department of Health, Education and Welfare has taken vital steps to improve reading skills within the United States by setting up the Office of Reading Disorders. It has encompassed two separate fields of study (a) the medical perspective and (b) the educational perspective. Thus, those children who cannot read can truly benefit from help . . . much needed help . . . we can forget labeling and begin the process of working together.

The Enduring Mystery of Dyslexia

Warren R. Young

WARREN R. YOUNG, formerly science and medicine editor of *Life*, is the author of the forthcoming book *The Mystery of Dyslexia*.

This strange and potentially devastating affliction prevents millions of otherwise bright children from learning to read or write normally. Yet it *can* be overcome

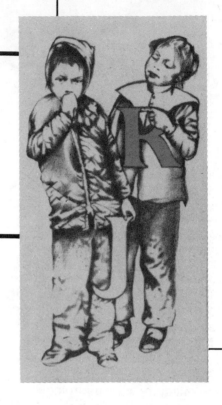

ONE CHILD in every seven has it, to some degree, often with tragic impact on his schooling and life. Up to three-quarters of juvenile delinquents may suffer from it, and careful studies suggest that it may be one of the most potent factors behind their rebellion. It probably kept inventor Thomas Edison, Gen. George S. Patton and President Woodrow Wilson from coping with ordinary schoolwork when they were young. It made Hans Christian Andersen an atrocious speller all his life, even though he became a magnificent storyteller. It most likely accounted for the nickname "Mr. Dullard," given a schoolboy named Albert Einstein.

The specific problem these people have in common is called dyslexia (from the Greek roots *dys*, "difficulty," and *lexia*, "pertaining to words"). Although it is unrelated to basic intellectual capacity, the affliction causes a mysterious difficul-ty in handling words and symbols. Some subtle peculiarity in the brain's organizational pattern blocks out an otherwise bright child's ability to learn how to read, to write legibly, to spell or, perhaps, to use numbers. Letters in words perversely transpose themselves, get reversed or even top-sy-turvy—"dog" becomes "god"; "b" changes identity with "d," and may even masquerade as "p" or "q"; a sign saying "OIL" flip-flops into "710." Many dyslexics also have difficulty orienting themselves in the three dimensions of space, which results, sometimes, in bodily awkwardness.

Ever since dyslexia was identified late in the 19th century by German and British ophthalmologists, it has been studied and debated. It is still an unsolved problem. Because it is unaccompanied by outward scars or detectable neurological damage, and because its bizarre symptoms vary from victim to victim, some professionals insist that the problem doesn't really exist as a separate entity. Educators in particular have shown a preference for herding this problem along with others under the broad, vaguely defined umbrella of "learning disabilities." Yet frustrated classroom teachers, agonized parents and humiliated victims know that *something*—something unique and devastating—is there.

Vice President Nelson A. Rockefeller is one of the most eminent dyslexics now living. "I often see letters and numbers backwards," he says, "or even think them backwards." A few lines from his boyhood diary, written when he was 11, include such revealing notations as "lunc," "picknick Lunch," "Uncil Harold," "engen repar schop," "parak" (for park), and three tries at recording the disease his sister Abby had come down with—"mealess," "measless" and "misless." Rockefeller never mastered spelling. Yet he graduated *cum laude* from Dartmouth Col-

"The Enduring Mystery of Dyslexia," Warren R. Young, *Reader's Digest*, Vol. 108 No. 646, February 1976. ©1975 Warren R. Young.

lege, and earned a Phi Beta Kappa key.

There was no secret cure behind Rockefeller's success in overcoming his handicap. The key was simply learning to cope. Coping to him meant concentrating very hard when something had to be read; even today, he lets aides fix up his spelling and he rehearses speeches carefully before delivering them.

Other dyslexics also achieved celebrity status by adapting to the realities of their difficulty. Woodrow Wilson did not learn the alphabet until he was nine, didn't read until he was 11, and was considered by relatives to be dull and backward. At Princeton University, his grades were only fair; but his brilliant oratorical style began to blossom at the same time, paving the way for his two distinguished Presidencies—of Princeton and of the United States.

General Patton had even harder sledding. At 12 he still could not read. It took him five years to get through West Point, and at that he made it only by laboriously memorizing his textbooks word for word.

Not all dyslexics are so fortunate, or so tenacious. Taunted by classmates, treated as lazy, stupid or mentally disturbed by teachers and parents, humiliated by schoolwork other children do so easily, many of them not only fail miserably in class but become filled with frustration, rage and pain. It is interesting to note that the telltale signs of the problem can be detected in the diary of Lee Harvey Oswald.

Trying to pin down the precise cause of dyslexia involves a number of basic riddles. How, really, do our minds work? How do we learn to read and write? How can an intelligent child—or even an adult creative genius—look straight at a word and interpret some of the letters backward, upside down or transposed? Why does the problem appear to turn up three times as often among boys as among girls? There are a dozen theories to explain dyslexia, but a final verdict is not yet in.

Ever since the turn of the century, one guess has been that defective vision must be to blame. This idea was based in part on the fact that poor readers employ inefficient eye movements. But experts now regard

---

Does Your Child Have Dyslexia?

YOUR child may need specialized help in overcoming the handicap of dyslexia if he or she shows some of these signs:

Reading difficulty; persistent spelling errors (especially misspelling the same familiar word different ways; reversed or upside-down letters, or reversed sequence of letters within words; uncertain preference for right- or left-handedness after age five or six; badly cramped, scrawled or illegible handwriting; confusion about left and right, up and down, tomorrow and yesterday; delayed mastery of spoken language, trouble finding the "right" word when talking; inadequacy in written composition; personal disorganization (losing or leaving possessions, inability to stick to simple schedules, repeatedly forgetting).

Few dyslexics show *all* these symptoms; and children who are not dyslexic may show some. But a pattern of these signs—especially a reading or spelling problem—means you would be wise to get a professional opinion. Talk with your child's teacher, school psychologist, learning-disabilities specialist or pediatrician as soon as possible, and request a full battery of diagnostic tests. If your child is definitely dyslexic, he or she will probably need careful, long-range one-to-one tutoring on a regular basis. But avoid signing up for remedial help—particularly any non-tutoring scheme—without first getting trustworthy expert advice.

For further information on dyslexia, write: The Orton Society, Inc., 8415 Bellona Lane, Towson, Md. 21204; or the Association for Children With Learning Disabilities, 5225 Grace St., Pittsburgh, Pa. 15236. Please enclose a stamped, self-addressed envelope.

---

faulty eye movements as the result, not the cause, of failure to recognize words. It is the brain, not the eye, that learns to read. So the question remains: what goes wrong in the brain?

Some early experts thought brain damage was responsible, since it was known that some victims of head injuries lost their reading and writing skills. But autopsies and brainwave studies tend to rule out injury as a common cause of dyslexia.

If detectable brain damage is not the cause, what about more subtle insults to the prenatal or infant brain? Some studies seem to show that lead in the air, physical trauma or oxygen deprivation during birth can sometimes affect language learning capability. However, careful tracings of family trees suggest that the problem may more often be a matter of heredity.

A sizable body of opinion clings to the "late-bloomer" theory, which holds that for no particular reason some children simply do not mature to the reading-readiness stage as early as others.

The theory that still probably comes closest to explaining dyslexia was developed some 50 years ago by Dr. Samuel Torrey Orton, then director of the Iowa State Psychopathic

Hospital. While screening mental-health problems, Orton became interested in children who not only repeatedly reversed letters or words, but had a talent for "mirror writing." Some of them could actually write better from right to left, with letters oriented backward and in reverse order, so that a mirror held alongside would show the words as they are normally written.

Orton knew that mirror writing came more naturally than regular writing for many left-handers or partial left-handers. Leonardo da Vinci, who was ambidextrous, often sketched with his right hand, while setting down notes mirror-fashion with his left. Orton, an expert neurologist, reasoned that while each half of the brain controls various natural activities, only one side becomes dominant in the use of language. If, in learning the artificial skill of recognizing symbols and translating them into words, both hemispheres persisted in taking part, they might somehow compete and interfere with each other, leading to reversed or jumbled perception. Orton concluded that it was not being left-handed that caused the problem, since many dyslexics are right-handed; rather, it was confused or mixed dominance of the brain's hemispheres.

1. DYSLEXIA – AN OVERVIEW

Fortunately, even the victim of severe, classic dyslexia can now learn, with the proper help, how to read at a decent speed and to write legibly. But parents should be wary. Still-unproven methods, as well as thoroughly discredited techniques, are also being offered, including everything from bouncing on trampolines and avoidance of food additives to psychotherapy and elaborate eye exercises.

The experts' consensus is that the best solution as of today is educational: careful, systematic, one-to-one tutoring on a regular basis to teach the dyslexic child the principles of phonics—the letter sounds which make up words. What the dyslexic child needs is to be shown how to decode the sounds for which single letters and combinations of letters stand, and how to fit them together into words. Since every dyslexic child's problems are different, individual tutoring techniques must also vary. Often, modern phonics specialists reinforce the child's familiarity with the shape of a letter or the sound of a word fragment by putting to work more than one of his senses. They might have a child look at a letter, say it aloud, trace its shape in the air and on the blackboard, feel a 3-D cutout of the letter. Once the skill of decoding (and the reverse process, encoding) is mastered, a child can read and write any word.

The encouraging prognosis for properly tutored dyslexics was firmly documented in a recent study by language consultant Margaret Byrd Rawson. She carefully followed a group of 20 boys with moderate to severe dyslexia, all of whom had been given structured, multi-sensory language training, to see exactly what happened after they grew up. All but one went to college; 18 earned degrees, then went on to obtain a total of 32 postgraduate degrees. Two became physicians, one a lawyer, two college professors, one a school principal, three teachers, two research scientists, three owners of businesses, three junior business executives, one an actor, one a skilled laborer and one a factory foreman.

Not all properly tutored dyslexics will do so well, of course. Yet it is also clear that dyslexics no longer need fail simply because of language problems.

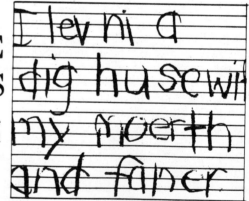

The Relationship of Reading Disabilities to Learning Disabilities

WINIFRED D. KIRK, M.A., Ph.B
University of Arizona

Janet Lerner has made a significant contribution to the field of learning disabilities (LD) in her article "Remedial Reading and Learning Disabilities: Are They the Same or Different?" Some differentiations she makes, however, may have opened a Pandora's box of disagreement between and within the two fields. The article outlines differences relating to "the nature of the problem, the label to be given to the phenomenon, the diagnostic procedures required, and the proposed treatment for the disorder" (p. 119 [of text]). Categorizing and oversimplifying the differences into two loosely defined fields of study may have created a spurious dichotomy and misrepresentation of both fields.

THE NATURE OF THE PROBLEM

In discussing the nature of the problem, Lerner has defined the area of mutual concern for both the reading specialist and members of the LD movement as "reading problems." This is a deceptive delineation since not all reading problems are of concern to the LD field. Problems resulting from poor teaching, emotional disturbance, poor school attendance, etc., are not directly due to learning disabilities, though they are reading problems. This distinction is important, for the LD specialist is concerned with intrinsic, not extrinsic, bases of the problem—whether they be in reading or in other areas. If remediation involves counteracting environmental influences rather than central processing difficulties (when such a distinction can be made), it is primarily the concern of the reading teacher. This distinction, of course, cannot be drawn until the diagnosis is made, whether the diagnostician calls himself a reading specialist or an LD specialist.

Lerner notes that in the field of reading two types of programs are differentiated: developmental and remedial reading. She states that remedial reading "designates programs for individuals who are not learning to read for a variety of reasons" (p. 120 [of text]). Many reading specialists and most authorities in LD make a finer differentiation, discriminating three types of reading: (a) developmental reading, which is the orderly development of reading skills; (b) corrective reading, which is involved in bringing a retarded reader up to his ability level by correcting or compensating for poor teaching, lack of school attendance, or other such detrimental experiences; and

(c) remedial reading (RR), which is teaching that takes into account the intrinsic difficulties of the child. (Harris, 1970; Kirk, 1966; Otto & McMenemy, 1966).

Not all authorities make this distinction between corrective and remedial reading; some use the term "remedial reading" to include any procedure used to bring a child up to his potential. The distinction is quite apparent, however, when one observes certain children who do not learn to read in spite of good teaching, good environmental influences, and corrective tutoring using the usual methods of developmental reading. For the child who does not have intrinsic difficulties in central processing or other complicated problems, the techniques used in developmental reading are easily extended to corrective reading. Thus, Lerner's statement could be changed as follows: "the reading specialist sees little if any difference between the principles or practices followed in remedial [substitute "corrective"] reading and the everyday instructional activities of a conscientious, creative classroom teacher" (p. 122 [of text]). In discussing RR, Lerner is not differentiating between the normal intact child who has missed some steps in the hierarchy of reading skills and the child with some intrinsic perceptual, cognitive, or intersensory difficulty. The problems cannot be oversimplified since most reading problems have at least an overlay of more than one element. The point I want to make is that when intrinsic deficiencies are related to a reading problem, these deficiencies must be taken into account and the teaching adapted to the problem.

A parallel situation exists in the area of oral language. Language arts are taught in the classroom as a developmental program. The teacher also deals with language problems from a corrective point of view for those children who have formed poor habits of language usage and who need special help in vocabulary, syntax, pronunciation, and so forth. But there are some children who need more specific help. The 6-year-old child, for example, who has little or no speech (but who is not mentally retarded, deaf, or autistic) can hardly receive adequate help in the classroom. He probably has an intrinsic difficulty in central processing and needs more exacting clinical teaching adapted to his intrinsic disability.

Lerner emphasizes another definition which has caused difficulty in communication: this is the term "dyslexia." She notes that it is ill-defined and misunderstood from person to person, that it conceals more than it reveals about the problem. Dr. Lerner, I believe, mistakenly attributes the use of this term to those in the field of LD, whereas it is used mostly by some physicians and optometrists, and by only a limited number of LD specialists. Many LD authorities have spoken out emphatically against its use. It is hardly realistic to isolate "scholars in the disciplines of education, psychology, and reading," as Lerner does on page 125, [of text] from the field of LD.

Since both LD and the field of reading are outgrowths of education and psychology, it creates a spurious dichotomy to place LD in contradistinction to RR or in contradistinction to "the disciplines of education, psychology, and reading." Such an oversimplification tends to misrepresent

both fields, for not all reading specialists maintain that the same methods used in developmental and/or corrective reading should and can be used for reading disabilities. Nor do all, or even a majority, of those in LD hold to the medical model of interpreting learning disabilities.

THE LABEL OF LEARNING DISABILITIES

Lerner has given an incomplete description of the field of LD. In 1963 when the term "learning disability" first became popular, it incorporated the area previously known as "perceptually handicapped," "brain damaged," "neurologically handicapped," and a host of other terms implying a neurological basis for abnormal behavior. But the term "learning disability" was not limited to such problems and was not meant to exlude those other learning problems and irregularities of cognitive style not necessarily implying a neurological underpinning. In fact, the term was adopted in an effort to place the emphasis on corrective measures for controlling behavior (including the act of learning) rather than on etiology and medical concerns.

Long before there was a name applied to the field of LD, psychologists, educators, and physicians were interested in the child with *a major psychological and/or neurological impediment to the development of language, memory, comprehension, perception, or other significant thought process, and which:* (a) *manifests itself in poor school achievement or in poor interpersonal communication;* (b) *creates wide discrepancies in the child's performance;* (c) *cannot be accounted for solely by sensory deficit, mental retardation, emotional disturbance, or lack of opportunity to learn.* Such an impediment, known today as a "specific learning disability," often manifests itself as a reading disability. Experts in RR have been taking such intrinsic disabilities into account since long before there was a field called "learning disabilities." Astute clinicians, whatever name they go by, are dealing with LD. Similarly, many adequately trained specialists in LD are also aware of the research, theory, and practices in the field

of reading. It is interesting to note that many of those now active in LD (including Janet Lerner and S. A. Kirk as well as the writer) came into the field by way of reading disabilities. Others who deal with LD came into the field by way of communication and language disorders.

Wiederholt (1974) outlines contributions to the field of LD as emanating from the study of disorders in spoken language, disorders of written language, and disorders of perceptual and motor processes. He states: "these three types of disorders were fairly separate until the birth of the field in 1963 .... Although medical professionals were responsible for the growth of the field during the foundation phase, psychologists during the transition phase, with educators currently holding major responsibilities for the rapid expansion during the integration phase, each profession continues to be represented in the field today" (p. 106). LD, young and somewhat nebulous, has not yet coalesced into a unified body of theory and practice. It is impossible to stereotype its members as representing one narrow point of view. In practice, this young field shows wide deviation in definition, in theory, in treatment, and in administrative procedures.

Because of its rapid expansion in the last 10 years, and because of the diversity of opinion within the field, a wide variety of children are being served by programs for the learning-disabled. Only recently did the federal and state governments subsidize assistance for LD, as they had earlier done for other handicaps. Because such state and federal funding has become available to many schools, while no well-defined demarcation has been made between reading disabilities and the educationally retarded child who does not show an intrinsic disability, both types of children are often being served by LD programs. Frequently, corrective service for minor reading deficiencies is not provided by local school systems, and therefore the federal and state funds are a boon to local reading programs. Also, much of the work being done under the caption of LD is corrective reading. A recent survey of programs (Elkins & Kirk, in press) indicates that a large proportion of children in LD programs are receiving assistance in reading and that a wide range of severity and correlated problems is included among them. In so far as the LD specialist moves into the field of corrective reading, he is further obfuscating any distinctiveness his own field possesses. It is most unfortunate that there are many "certified learning disabilities specialists" actively involved in LD programs who are not themselves experts in the field of reading.

TASK ANALYSIS—ITS PLACE IN DIAGNOSIS

Another difference of opinion which Lerner discusses is the use of task analysis as a diagnostic procedure. She notes that in the field of reading "the focus is on the subject matter rather than on assumed underlying processes" (p. 127 [of text]). While "in the field of LD, task analysis evaluates and analyzes the processing abilities required of a child to understand and perform a task (p. 126 [of text]). Here, again, terminology is a stumbling block to understanding possible differences between the two fields. Task analysis may be used in conjunction with diagnosis, but it is not a diagnostic procedure in and of itself. It is an analysis of the *what* that is to be taught. In Lerner's own words, "[the behavioral] approach to task analysis concentrates on operational analysis of a task to state specific behavioral objectives so that learning experiences can be designed to direct a child to reach these objectives" (1971, p. 73). Similarly Bateman defines task analysis as "the process of isolating, describing and sequencing . . . all necessary sub-tasks which, when the child has mastered them, will enable

him to perform the objective" (1971, p.33).

In LD, task analysis is a necessary element in the teaching process, and much is being borrowed from the behavioral approach. Tasks are analyzed, not only from the point of view of what subtasks are required for an orderly development of reading, but also from the point of view of what alternatives are possible in the manner of presentation and what mode of response is required of the child. The main difference comes in the added analysis of the child's abilities and disabilities and the correlates of the problem so as to understand the *how* of teaching in addition to the *what* that is to be taught. In order to understand why a child is having difficulty accomplishing a certain step in the hierarchy of skills, it is helpful to know where his weaknesses lie. We need not only the *what,* but also the *how* of learning. We need *child analysis* as well as *task analysis* in order to make a match between the two.

If a child cannot readily associate a sound with a visual symbol or a word, the LD specialist wants to know whether it is because the child lacks a visual image of the symbol or the word, or because he cannot re-auditorize the sound or the words, or because he is slow in intersensory paired-associate learning, or because he has difficulty making such responses automatic. An adept and experienced teacher may be able to recognize what process leads to the difficulty and may prevent problems if she is aware of the possible pitfalls. For some less perceptive teachers or less experienced teachers, more organized methods of determining the basis of the difficulty may be needed. The subskills of word attack, study methods, com-

2. Reading/Learning Disabilities

prehension, etc., become important as devices for determining the child's attainment; but the child's intrinsic deficits may determine how the next step is accomplished. For developmental reading and corrective reading, this requirement is not as demanding as it is in the hard-core reading disability cases.

A FORWARD LOOK

Perhaps the two fields are not as far apart as appears on the surface. It may be mainly a difference of emphasis. A successful behavioral approach emphasizes the analysis of the task but also, perhaps incidentally, evaluates the child's faltering steps in order to know where to zero in and materialize on the child's learning processes. It is often possible to improve the weak areas through appropriate methods of teaching the child to read.

Actually, Lerner has brought to our attention several differences which not only cross fields but also hold within each field. Elkins (1974) has pointed out that in Australia the conflict between LD and reading problems does not exist, since they both fit into a single administrative system. The dichotomy between fields may be spurious, but real issues are at stake. As Lerner has stated in her epilogue, "in the real world the demarcation is not so clear. Operationally the two fields may be quite similar. . . . It seems important to recast both fields by searching for a higher framework of synthesis—one that takes into account both systems of studying and treating reading problems" (pp. 179–183 [of text]). Janet Lerner is eminently qualified to pursue this framework and show the other side of the coin—the integrative possibilities of the two fields.

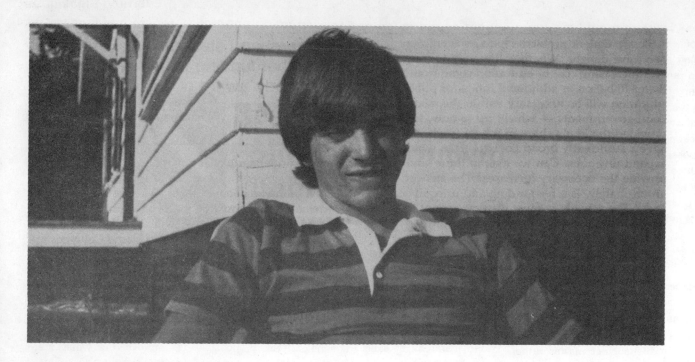

On Being Seventeen, Bright — and Unable to Read

By David Raymond

One day a substitute teacher picked me to read aloud from the textbook. When I told her "No, thank you," she came unhinged. She thought I was acting smart, and told me so. I kept calm, and that got her madder and madder. We must have spent 10 minutes trying to solve the problem, and finally she got so red in the face I thought she'd blow up. She told me she'd see me after class.

Maybe someone like me was a new thing for that teacher. But she wasn't new to me. I've been through scenes like that all my life. You see, even though I'm 17 and a junior in high school, I can't read because I have dyslexia. I'm told I read "at a fourth-grade level," but from where I sit, that's not reading. You can't know what that means unless you've been there. It's not easy to tell how it feels when you can't read your homework assignments or the newspaper or a menu in a restaurant or even notes from your own friends.

My family began to suspect I was having problems almost from the first day I started school. My father says my early years in school were the worst years of his life. They weren't so good for me, either. As I look back on it now, I can't find the words to express how bad it really was. I wanted to die. I'd come home from school screaming, "I'm dumb. I'm dumb — I wish I were dead!"

I guess I couldn't read anything at all then — not even my own name — and they tell me I didn't talk as good as other kids. But what I remember about those days is that I couldn't throw a ball where it was supposed to go, I couldn't learn to swim, and I wouldn't learn to ride a bike, because no matter what anyone told me, I knew I'd fail.

I just felt dumb. And dumb was how the kids treated me.

Sometimes my teachers would try to be encouraging. When I couldn't read the words on the board they'd say, "Come on, David, you know that word." Only I didn't. And it was embarrassing. I just felt dumb. And dumb was how the kids treated me. They'd make fun of me every chance they got, asking me to spell "cat" or something like that. Even if I know how to spell it, I wouldn't; they'd only give me another word. Anyway, it was awful, because more than anything I wanted friends. On my birthday when I blew out the candles I didn't wish I could learn to read; what I wished for was that the kids would like me.

With the bad reports coming from school, and with me moaning about wanting to die and how everybody hated me, my parents began looking for help. That's when the testing started. The school tested me, the child-guidance center tested me, private psychiatrists tested me. Everybody knew something was wrong — especially me.

It didn't help much when they stuck a fancy name onto it. I couldn't pronounce it then — I was only in second grade — and I was ashamed to talk about it. Now it rolls off my tongue, because I've been living with it for a lot of years — dyslexia.

All through elementary school it wasn't easy. I was always having to do things that were "different," things the other kids didn't have to do. I had to go to a child psychiatrist, for instance.

One summer my family forced me to go to a camp for children with reading problems. I hated the idea, but the camp turned out pretty good, and I had a good time. I met a lot of kids who couldn't read and somehow that helped. The director of the camp said I had a higher I.Q. than 90 percent of the population. I didn't believe him.

I'm told I read "at a fourth-grade level," but from where I sit, that's not reading.

About the worst thing I had to do in fifth and sixth grade was go to a special education class in another school in our town. A bus picked me up, and I didn't like that at all. The bus also picked up emotionally disturbed kids, and retarded kids. It was like going to a school for the retarded. I always worried that someone I knew would see me on that bus. It was a relief to go to the regular junior high school.

Life began to change a little for me then, because I began to feel better about myself. I found the teachers cared; they had meetings about me and I worked harder for them for a while. I began to work on the potter's wheel, making vases and pots that the teachers said were pretty good. Also, I got a letter for being on the track team. I could always run pretty fast.

At high school the teachers are good and everyone is trying to help me. I've gotten honors some marking period and I've won a letter on the cross country team. Next quarter I think the school might hold a show of my pottery. I've got some friends. But there are still some embarrasing times. For instance, every time there is writing in the class, I get up and go to the special education room. Kids ask me where I go all the time. Sometimes I say "to Mars."

Homework is a real problem. During free periods in school I go into the special ed room and staff members read assignments to me. When I get home my mother reads to me. Sometimes she reads an assignment into a tape recorder, and then I go into my room and listen to it. If we have a novel or something like that to read, she reads it out loud to me. Then I sit down with her and we do the assignment. She'll write, while I talk my answers to her. Lately I've taken to dictating into a tape recorder, and then someone — father, a private tutor or my mother — types up what I've dictated. Whatever homework I do takes someone else's time, too. That makes me feel bad.

We had a big meeting in school the other day — eight of us, four from the guidance department, my private tutor, my parents and me. The subject was me. I said I wanted to go to college, and they told me about colleges that have facilities and staff to handle people like me. That's nice to hear.

As for what happens after college, I don't know and I'm worried about that. How can I make a living if I can't read? Who will hire me? How will I fill out the application form? The only thing that gives me any courage is the fact that I've learned about well-known people who couldn't read or had other problems and still made it. Like Albert Einstein, who didn't talk until he was 4 and flunked math. Like Leonardo da Vinci, who everyone seems to think had dyslexia.

I've told this story because maybe some teacher will read it and go easy on a kid in the classroom who has what I've got. Or, maybe some parent will stop nagging his kid, and stop calling him lazy. Maybe he's not lazy or dumb. Maybe he just can't read and doesn't know what's wrong. Maybe he's scared, like I was.

Dyslexia: What you can—and can't—do about it

There are no easy answers to helping the dyslexic child. But there are more effective approaches to the problem than simply ignoring it. Here's what a noted neurologist advises.

R.M.N. CROSBY, M.D. with ROBERT A. LISTON

About the authors: *Dr. R. M. N. Crosby is a pediatric neurologist and neurosurgeon in Baltimore. Robert A. Liston is author of numerous articles and books.*

I**N NEARLY EVERY** grade school classroom there is a child or two and in slow learning classes many youngsters who are dyslexic. They seem intelligent. They want to read. But for seemingly inexplicable reasons they just "don't get the hang of it." The dyslexic child is slow to learn to read in the first grade, and he continues to lag behind until by the upper elementary grades he is a year or more behind grade level.

We are not suggesting that every problem reader is dyslexic. There are many causes for reading disorders, including children who are idle, lack intelligence, have emotional problems, are culturally deprived or have been poorly taught. Teachers are familiar with these problems and accustomed to assisting such pupils in any way they can.

There is another major cause for reading difficulties—brain dysfunction—which, in its various forms, makes it difficult for the child to learn to read. Through no fault of theirs, teachers are simply less familiar with neurological reading disorders and are thereby less able to help the child. If blame must be assessed, it must lie with neurologically trained physicians who have known and diagnosed these brain impairments for over 50 years, yet have not communicated this information to other medical specialities, let alone teachers, psychologists and parents.

Our book, *The Waysiders* (Delacorte) sought to bridge this information gap with sufficient information to enable the layman, in general, and teachers, in particular, to recognize the dyslexic child and cope with the extremely difficult educational problem he poses. We suggested in the book that teachers needed to become aware of the nature of the dyslexic's neurological impairments, learn to identify the dyslexic youngster from among the various problem readers, arrange to have his impairment diagnosed . . . and then begin to find ways to teach him. We felt, and still feel, that this is a bit much for a classroom teacher with 25 or more pupils demanding attention. We urged her, and still do, to seek the help of the school psychologist, neurologically trained physician, and remedial reading instructor.

This is the ideal approach. But the fact is that the overwhelming majority of teachers do not have expert assistance available. They are "going it alone" in coping with the neurologically impaired child. And they need practical information to help them educate a dyslexic child.

This article has been written to partially fill that need. We hope it will help you understand the nature of dyslexia and why it is so educationally debilitating to the child. We hope it will help you recognize the dyslexic child among other types of problem readers and perhaps identify some of the more common impairments, so an educational program can be planned. *But more than anything else, we hope you will come to understand the desperate plight of the dyslexic child and why his really very minor impairments are so psychologically destructive.*

The human brain is not stamped out by a machine. No two of us are alike in our neurological capacities. We all have brain dysfunctions of which we are either unaware or which we look upon as idiosyncrasies. Some of us have poor depth perception or an inferior sense of direction or below average coordination. Our abilities to perceive colors or sounds or rhythms may be less sharp than others, and some of us are color blind and tone deaf. There are many, many such dysfunctions, each varying from total incapacity to simple slowness to learn.

"Dyslexia: What You Can – And Can't – Do About It," R.M.N. Crosby, M.D., with Robert A. Liston, *A Grade Teacher Notebook*, 1969.

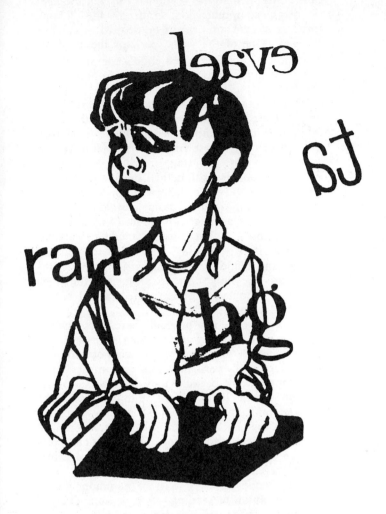

"His eyesight may be 20/20, yet he cannot perceive minute differences in the shapes of letters. If his impairment is serious, he won't be able to tell the difference between a letter and a number. He won't learn the alphabet, let alone read."

The dyslexic child is no different than the rest of us. He has extremely minor impairments in his ability to perceive shapes and sounds. But in his case, the impairments are highly debilitating, for they make it difficult for him to learn to read and write. Since our entire educational system, with one or two exceptions, is geared to learning by reading, the dyslexic child is denied an education and all the economic and cultural rewards that stem therefrom.

Consider the dyslexic child. He appears to be normal. He is intelligent, often extremely intelligent, with great capacity to learn. He does not limp, stutter, wear thick spectacles. He is profi-

cient at baseball, a great teller of tales, a marvelous friend, everything boys and girls are everywhere—until he goes to school. Then he faces the first and biggest failure of his life. He has trouble learning to read.

He *wants* to learn. He tries as hard as he can, but nothing seems to work. Everyone else in the class is learning. Why isn't he? He becomes acutely conscious of his failure. He is buried somewhere in the third reading group. His efforts at oral reading are accompanied by titters from his classmates and sometimes the criticism of his teacher. He takes home a report card that looks like an exercise in the lower letters of the alphabet.

His parents are disapppointed, accuse him of lazinesss, take away privileges until he improves his grades and often corporally punish him. In time, he may be tested by the school psychologist, examined by doctors and banished to remedial reading. He fails grades and becomes a 10-year-old third-grader, the big dumb kid. He gives up on education, school, his parents and himself. Who can fail to understand that this child must find something he's good at—perhaps sports, perhaps only mischief and trouble making?

Many such youngsters come to the pediatric neurologist's office. They sit there—sullen, defeated, their potential wasted. One who comes particularly to mind was a 13-year-old fifth-grader. He had been picked up by police for shoplifting from a drug store. Juvenile officers realized that there was something "wrong" with him and asked school officials to investigate. When a psychologist, social worker and pediatrician failed to find any cause for his school difficulty, he was referred for neurological examination.

This young man had an IQ of 113, yet he was an abysmal school failure. His teacher reported: "This child doesn't like school. He doesn't pay attention in class. His mind wanders, and he looks out the window. I can't blame him for that, for he still reads at the first grade level. Actually, he doesn't even know the alphabet. He is poor in arithmetic. He will fail again this year."

1. DYSLEXIA – AN OVERVIEW

Records showed the boy had failed the first, second and third grades. His explanation for his ability to pass the fourth grade was, "They had to paint the classroom." He sat in the office quite sullen and uncommunicative. Yet, when asked what he would like to do more than anything else in the world, he replied, "I want to read."

Neurological examination showed why he had not read. He had a severe disorder of visual perception, performing at age 13 about as well as a seven-year-old. He also had poor tactile perception.

Such a child is a serious problem. He is a problem to the neurologist, who is in the difficult position of being able to diagnose, but not "cure" or even treat him. There are no pills, injections or surgical techniques. It is the measure of the problem that the only one who can "treat" him is his teacher.

At the same time, we cannot blame the teacher for failing to recognize this—or any other—dyslexic child. The dyslexic child often looks like every other problem reader. If he doesn't seem intelligent, it is simply because having read less he knows less. It is not uncommon to find dyslexic children in classes for the mentally retarded. As the boy described above, he seems lazy. But why should he work? It isn't getting him anywhere. He has emotional problems stemming from his frustration, embarrassment and ridicule. He is culturally deprived because of the reading problem he has.

And so, this child, in the vast majority of cases, goes unrecognized, untaught. He becomes a casualty of education, falling by the wayside in the thrust for learning and all its benefits—and all because of neurological idiosyncrasies such as we all may have.

The teacher who wishes to recognize and aid dyslexic children, needs to have some understanding of reading as a neurological process. A neurologist looks at reading somewhat differently than an educator, and understanding this difference is vital to teaching the dyslexic child.

All learning is a function of the brain—but different functions. Much of what a child (or any person) learns in or out of school involves a brain function which might be called *comprehension*. He understands the meaning of oral speech and of many signs, symbols, gestures and facial expressions by which meaning is conveyed. If he is not dyslexic and learns to read, he comprehends the meaning of printed words. There are many other brain functions involved in education, including *memory* and *recall,* but going into these here will lead us rather far afield. What is important is for you to realize that comprehension is *one* function of the brain. If a child has very much of a dysfunction in comprehension, he simply is never going to appear in a regular classroom. He doesn't even understand speech. He is retarded.

Nearly everything taught in school, including history, geography, science, all the information and concepts man has compiled through the ages, involves comprehension. Indeed, the lifelong process of education might be defined as comprehension. One of the ways, perhaps the most important way, you increase a child's comprehension is by teaching him to read—a different function of the brain.

This is not playing with words. There is an area (or areas) of the brain which has the function of language comprehension. There is another area (or areas) whose function is reading. There are others whose function is writing, still others whose function is arithmetical calculation. When you teach a child to read, to write or to calculate, you are teaching him a basic neurological function which is in a direct continuum of rolling over, reaching and grasping, sitting, standing, walking, climbing stairs, running, talking and training bowels and bladder. Reading, writing and arithmetic are the only basic neurological functions taught in school. All others were learned before the child came to school.

Two points need to be made here. First, we all understand that there are children with perfectly formed vocal apparatus who cannot talk or youngsters with normal bones and musculature who cannot walk because they have a neurological impairment. It should not be difficult to accept the fact that there are youngsters who have difficulty in reading, writing and calculation because of neurological impairment. The significant difference is that the former are grossly observable, while the latter are hard to detect.

The second point is that the common educational definition of reading—that is, obtaining the meaning from or bringing meaning to the printed word—complicates an already complex process by confusing the function of comprehension with the function of reading.

What is reading then? From a neurological standpoint, *reading is translating graphic symbols into SOUND according to a recognized system.* When a child enters the first grade, he has an oral vocabulary variously estimated at between 2,500 and 20,000 words, depending upon his intelligence, his maturity and the environment to which he has been exposed. His neurological network is well established; the sound of a word, received by his ear and converted into nerve impulses, is sent to the area or areas of the brain whose function is comprehension.

Now, the child arrives at school. You write the word "run" on the blackboard. You say the word aloud. The child knows the oral word *run.* He has heard it thousands of times. You are saying to him that those three letters are simply a written expression of that word he has heard so many times and knows so well. What the child does, in the beginning, is add a sight link to his existing pattern for oral speech.

In a rather short time—if he is not dyslexic—the child goes to a second level of reading wherein the sight of a word automatically tells him its sound and thus its meaning. He hears mentally; he may actually say the word silently to himself setting up measurable vibrations in his vocal cords. With practice, he becomes quite rapid at the translation of sight to sound.

Most people read at this second level throughout life. It is a perfectly acceptable, even advantageous way to read, although somewhat slower. A few people go to a third level, establishing an entirely new network so that the sight of a word automatically triggers its meaning. Its sound is eliminated.

Many people cannot learn to read this way no matter how hard they try. It is certainly not something to be taught in the primary grades.

Reading, then, is translating marks on paper into sound according to a recognized system. Translating marks on paper into sound requires the ability to recognize the letters of the written alphabet and the sounds they represent. In English, this is grossly difficult. The letters are amazingly similar. Reversals are common— *b, d, p, q* and, if the handwriting is imprecise, *h* and *g; m, w* and *3; z, N, s, 2* and *5; a* and *e; c* and *u*.

The array of sounds those letters and combinations of them make, together with the confusing, often bizarre spelling patterns of the language, make reading so difficult that one would not believe it possible if so many didn't do it. That so many learn to read is certainly a tribute to the genius of children and their teachers!

Now consider dyslexia. Dyslexia is not a disease. It is a disability resulting from brain dysfunctions of various types, but predominantly impairment of visual or auditory perception. Visual perception enables person to recognize the differences and similarities between shapes and forms. By visual perception, a person can detect the difference between a triangle and a square and the similarities between an *A* and, say, the shape of a tent's end. Auditory perception is the ability to detect similarities

and differences between sounds, such as *leaf* and *leave* or music played in a different key.

Teachers should be acquainted with a third type of perception, for reasons to be made clear shortly. We refer to tactile perception, the ability to recognize the differences and similarities in shape and pattern by touch alone.

If you as a teacher realize that a child can read because he can recognize the letters in the English language and the sounds they make, then you will be able to understand the difficulty of a child

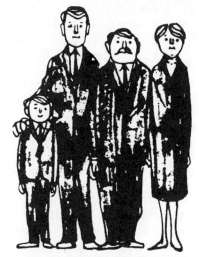

In one out of four cases there is a genetic basis to dyslexia.

who has impairment in visual or auditory perception. His eyesight may be 20/20, yet he cannot perceive those minute differences in the shapes of letters. If his impairment is serious, he won't be able to tell the difference between a letter and a number. He won't even learn the alphabet, let alone read. If he has auditory imperception, that array of phonic sounds is his Mount Everest. If he has anything other than a very slight auditory imperception, you as a teacher will never get to meet him, for he has never learned to understand or speak a language. Hopefully, he will go to a school for the aphasic child.

Your first problem as a teacher is to identify the dyslexic child from among that array of problem readers you have. There are sev-

eral characteristics of dyslexia which may be helpful to you.

First, he can read *some.* We have seen some extremely serious dyslexics, but we have seen few children who did not learn to read at least a little.

Second, in this article we are referring to the mild to moderate impairment. To repeat, if he has any more than a slight auditory imperception, he won't be in school. If he has a moderate to serious visual imperception, he will stand out in kindergarten and the first grade. He won't know a letter from a number, a triangle from a circle. Reading at this time will be totally out of the question. The child with the mild to moderate imperception is the one we described earlier. He is slow to learn. He lags behind and by the fourth or fifth grade he is one to three years behind grade level. He is also the fellow you are apt to be coping with.

Third, dyslexia occurs four to five times more frequently among boys than girls. The reasons for this are little understood.

Fourth, in about one quarter of the cases, dyslexia is genetic in origin. If the boy has had siblings, parents, grandparents or aunts and uncles with reading problems, you may look upon this as a clue to the *A-ha!* variety. But remember, dyslexia occurs without any genetic origins, too.

Fifth, dyslexia has some relationship to left-handedness. This is a thorny neurological thicket that it is impossible for us to go into in this article. But there is a significantly greater percentage of left handedness in neurologically impaired readers than in the general population. Do not be confused by the concept of crossed or mixed dominance (right eyed, left handed, etc.). This has nothing to do with reading disability. The distribution of so-called mixed dominance is the same in the neurologically impaired readers as it is in superior readers. The clue here is not to suspect all left-handed children, but to suspect a neurological basis for the difficulty in a left-handed poor reader.

Sixth, in a significant, but unknown percentage of cases, dyslexia tends to be maturational. A boy who has gross impairment in the first and second grades may, but will not necessarily, show marked improvement as he nears puberty. There will undoubtedly be *some* improvement with age. This characteristic of dyslexia should be of particular interest to you. We have seen many, many children who had severe perceptual impairments at age six or seven. Teaching them to read at that time was extremely difficult, requiring extended one-to-one instruction. Yet, by age 10 or 12 their impairment had improved so that teaching them to read would be much easier. Trouble is, the child was so psychologically scarred by his educational experience that he no longer wanted to learn. He'd given up on education. Your major task as a teacher is to prevent that psychological scarring from occurring.

Seventh, each dyslexic child is unique. That is the staggering aspect of the educational problem. His perceptual impairments may occur with various other neurological deficiencies or they may not. His impairments can range from severe to mild. Infinite variety is possible. Thus, the educational problem is that the educational program for the dyslexic—and he can be taught—must be tailored to fit his individual needs. Thus, the child should have careful diagnosis that pinpoints the nature and extent of his impairments.

Can you as a teacher diagnose dyslexia? Ideally, no. A neurologically trained physician or psychologist should do it. But as a practical matter, we would far rather have an informed teacher take a stab at it than nothing be done. But let's make a deal: you won't practice medicine and we won't teach school, an expertise in which we are entirely unqualified. There are complexities and subtleties to dyslexia which require neu-

rological training. *But there is no reason why you can't learn to detect the forms of imperception which are most commonly seen.*

The first step in any diagnosis is the observation that the child reads at least a year behind grade level for his age. If he reads at grade level, he is no reading problem, no matter how much you might think him an underachiever. As a practical matter, the dyslexic child will read two or more years below grade level. In the first grade, he will quickly fall behind his classmates. If he has even a moderate impairment, you will undoubtedly recommend that he repeat the grade.

The second step is to have the suspect child read aloud. This is where you will have your mettle tested. Among the cleverest human beings I have ever seen are intelligent dyslexic children. They read—somehow, from context, from pictures, from smudge marks on the page, from people's expressions as they listen, anyway, everyway. I had a patient, quite a severe dyslexic, who had her mother convinced that she was an expert reader until one day the mother caught her reading aloud from a book that was upside down.

Listen to the child read. It is imperative that you be alone; just the two of you. Select some material that the child has never seen before. Take it out of context, such as the middle of a page. Make sure there are no pictures that will tell what the material is about.

Have the child read aloud while you listen as carefully as you can, comparing what he reads to the text. In all probability, what he reads will make sense. He'll get the meaning. His will be a case of almost, but not quite. An intelligent child with mild dyslexia will misread individual words (*begins* for *beginning* for example). He'll slur words to mask what he's saying. If you correct him, he'll insist that is what he said. He'll be slow and very careful. If his impairment is a little greater, he'll make apparently senseless substitutions,

such as *train* for *taught* or *music* for *marry*.

Step three. Observe his writing, for the dyslexic child is often more readily detected through his spelling than his reading. The reason is simple. He can fake and fudge reading, but when he writes he is entirely on his own. The medical term for the inability to write (more correctly *spell*) is *dysgraphia*. The dyslexic child almost invariably is also dysgraphic because of his perceptual impairments. Figure 1 (page 83) is an example of dysgraphia produced by a 10-year-old. On the left are his efforts. On the right are the corrections made by his teacher. Figure 2 is the spelling paper of a 12-year-old girl in the fifth grade. No one would consider these simply poor spellers. On most of the words, they are not even close, and what they have written, although legible, makes no sense. The dyslexic child in your class will differ from these only in degree.

We also suggest that you have the child copy some material, something out of a book or something you have written for him. Copying is much easier for the child than making sentences up out of his head. Any errors in spelling or malformations of letters should give you a strong indication of dyslexia.

Step four. What you have done so far may enable you to suspect that the child is dyslexic. You will be doing the child, yourself and his parents a big favor if you can discover *why* he has this symptom. Does he have auditory or visual imperception . . . or both?

Auditory imperception is seen far less often and is difficult to detect. We suggest that you listen to the child's speech carefully. He

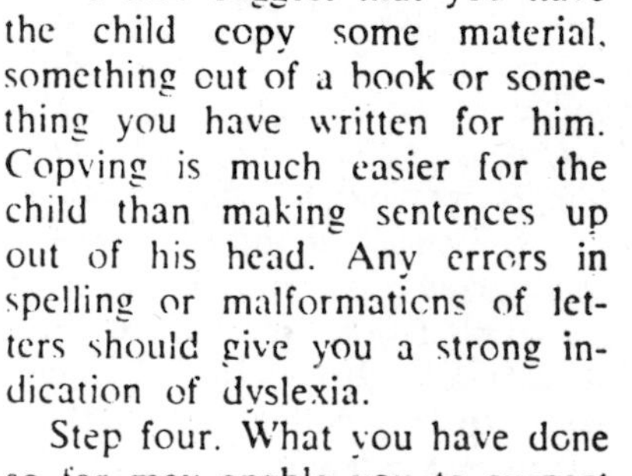

Fig. 1

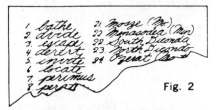

Two examples of dysgraphia: Fig. 1 by a 10-year-old boy; fig. 2 by a 12-year-old girl patient.

will make a few substitutions of sounds on a fairly regular basis, such as an *h* sound for a *p* sound or an *f* sound for a *b* sound.

His speech will not have the characteristics of a speech impediment. His diction will be good, but what he says will be incomprehensible. One illustration: A 12-year-old girl relegated to classes for the mentally retarded because she had lapsed into nearly total silence, finally volunteered that her favorite television program was "Fatman." When we said we were unfamiliar with the program, she said, with some irritation, "You know, the man who looks like a *fat* and has the little boy with him." She meant, of course, *Batman.*

Visual imperception is the impairment you will encounter most frequently, and in the detection of this you may be somewhat more scientific. We test visual perception by means of the Bender-Gestalt drawing, produced in Figure 3 (page 84). This is a sophisticated test which enables the tester to measure and grade a child's performance according to his age with a high degree of accuracy. Unless you have had some training, it is unlikely that you will be able to make accurate measurements, but there is no reason you can't use the test to detect visual imperception in a broad sense. Figure 4 is an example of a very poor test performance by a kindergarten child. Observe the quite terrible spatial relationships in items *A*, *4* and *8*. Figure 5 is a test which ordinarily wouldn't be considered too bad, except that the person is 27 years old, has a verbal IQ of 135 and can't read at all. The test

Fig. 3

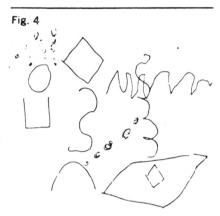

Fig. 4

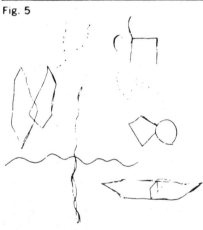

Fig. 5

Fig. 6

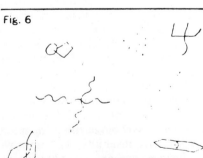

Bender-Gestalt drawing (top) and the attempts of three dyslexics to duplicate it.

indicates he could now learn, if he makes the effort. Figure 6 illustrates the test result of a 10-year-old, mildly dyslexic boy.

We recommend the Bender-Gestalt test to teachers who want some evidence of possible dyslexia in a student. It isn't an absolute essential, however. You can make a test of your own. Use simple forms, such as a circle inside a square so it touches all four sides or letter-like forms, combining curved and straight lines.

We also suggest you test the child's tactile perception. One way to do this is to have the child close his eyes and extend his hand. Then, using a paper clip or similar object, trace a number on one of his finger pads. Have him identify the number you have drawn, then draw another number on another pad and have the child identify it. Repeat the process, being sure to test both the child's hands. If he has tactile imperception, you will get various responses—including that of a child who can't identify any numbers unless they are traced very large on the palm of his hand, and who may even miss those. In less severe cases, you will get reversals.

We recommend that you go a step further. Instead of having the child identify aloud what you have traced, ask him to write it on a piece of paper. When we traced the figures of the fingerpads of the child who drew Figure 4, he failed completely. Then the figures were drawn two inches high on the palm of his hand. He reversed the 3 into an *M*. In two tries, the closest he could come to a + was an elongated *P*. In two tries at duplicating a triangle, he produced something resembling a Bedouin lean-to (in a state of disrepair). This child had a severe case of both tactile and visual imperception.

We realize that none of these diagnostic efforts are very easy. The results will not always be definitive. There are several other, less common learning disorders which will not be revealed. We are aware, too, that there are other causes for reading problems and that normal children make reversals and spell incomprehensibly. The dyslexic child simply makes more errors and persists in them longer than the normal child.

If you feel you have diagnosed a dyslexic child in your class, what can you do as a teacher? A great, great deal—but what you can do *least* well, in our opinion, is teach him to read. We don't mean that you lack the capacity. We simply fail to see how a teacher with 25 or more students can find the time to provide the intensive, individualized, extremely patient instruction needed by the dyslexic child.

But here are some recommendations in case you want to try. From a neurological standpoint, there are only three routes into language comprehension—the visual, the auditory and/or the tactile. In simplest terms, if one of those pathways is blocked by a perceptual impairment, effort should be concentrated upon those pathways that work. Which is to say: Teach to strengths, not to weakness.

If a child has visual imperception, it is cruelty to teach him to read by the whole word or look-say method. Better results will be achieved through phonics or kinesthetic methods, such as drawing in sand, feeling plastic letters or fashioning them from pipe cleaners. Obviously, if the child also has tactile imperception, the kinesthetic methods will only compound his frustration. If he has auditory imperception, phonics will be a mistake. We believe that a diagnosis of a child's perceptual disorders is vital to the development of a program that teaches him individually or in small groups.

Any remedial reading will be of *some* benefit to him. If possible, get him into such a program. Individual tutoring, if only a few minutes a day, is best. We have seen some amazing results from such a little effort, particularly when the tutor understands the child's impairment and makes use of his abilities.

A case in point is the 13-year-old shoplifter described earlier. A sympathetic teacher in his school volunteered to work with him during lunch hour. For 45 minutes a day, five days a week, she patiently taught him the shapes of letters and, stressing phonics to make use of his excellent auditory perception, gradually taught him to read. At the end of a year, he knew 300 words. After two years, he read at grade level. His entire attitude towards himself and school changed. Juvenile officers have forgotten about this child.

Whether you ever improve the child's reading, you have, as his teacher, a two-fold responsibility to him. The ultimate tragedy of the dyslexic child—or any problem reader for that matter—is that he is denied information. The aim of education is not to learn to read, after all, but to teach information and concepts. Reading is just one means to this end. A person could conceivably learn everything aurally, and lead a productive life. There are many occupations and professions that require only minimal reading, if only a person possesses information.

We are not suggesting that you turn your class upside down by reverting to an oral method of instruction. That would not be fair to the children who *can* read and *need* to read. But we are suggesting that whenever possible you encourage the dyslexic child to learn through movies, television, other visual aids, records, lectures, field trips and listening to class recitations. If at all possible, you should enlist the cooperation of his parents.

Your second responsibility is to see to it that the child is not ruined psychologically. In many cases, his disability will improve with age, perhaps disappearing altogether. It is vital that he not be soured on education, himself and life by the time that occurs.

The dyslexic child needs affection, approval and acceptance. He needs to know that he is a fine person, an intelligent person and not dumb in any sense of the word. He needs to know that he has fine qualities and abilities, but he happens to have a neurological idiosyncrasy that makes it more difficult for him to read and write. He needs to know that he will have to work harder and that he will often have to be satisfied with fewer results. He needs to know, despite this, that he has a future, that there are many areas of employment and real accomplishment available to him.

The dyslexic child needs to be protected from the ridicule of his classmates. He needs to read aloud, but *not* amidst destructive snickering. We believe you are the key person here. If you treat the child as the fine, intelligent person he really is, his classmates will too.

We believe that once you are aware of the dyslexic child's impairments, you will find it easier to make allowances for his poor handwriting, inferior spelling, and the slow pace of his reading. We hope you will be able to allow him more time, demand less of him, make allowances for his intent, and even find time to test him orally to confirm that *he knows information even though he can't write it on a test paper*.

The program we have suggested here is only stopgap. With three to four million dyslexic youngsters entering the first grade each year, even your best efforts are simply a finger in the dike of an immense and largely unrecognized educational problem. We hope that you, as a teacher, can raise your voice with ours, urging principals, superintendents, special education supervisors, boards of education and citizens generally to begin the educational efforts dyslexic children require and deserve.

Dyslexia: A Sure Cure

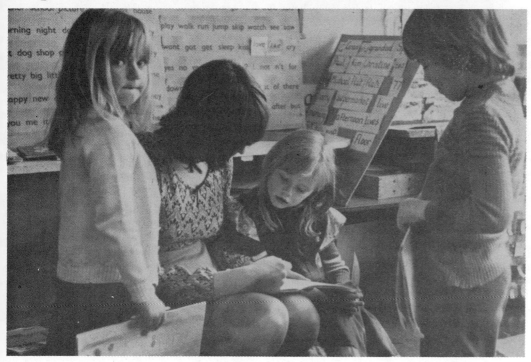

Frank W. Freshour

Dr. Freshour is Assistant Professor, Reading Education, University of South Florida, Tampa, Florida.

So Johnny cannot read and you are not making much progress in trying to teach him. If you are like many other teachers, you refer him to a public school reading clinic, to a private reading clinic or to a nearby university reading clinic if you are that fortunate. Oh yes, on the school information form which asks the nature of the reading problem you write "Dyslexia." That lets everyone off the hook, child, parent, teacher, and school alike. Certainly no one can be held responsible if the child has "Dyslexia." Now the experts get a shot at him. Unfortunately, it is because of these experts, the university reading professors, the private reading clinicians, the psychologists, the ophthalmologists, the pediatricians, and the neurologists that the child has "Dyslexia" in the first place. Teachers did not coin the term. Neither did parents nor children.

One of the reasons the term is in use today is that many of the self-proclaimed experts began to misuse it and thus are able to operate today under the umbrella of "Dyslexia." Other terms which are in vogue and fall under this nebulous umbrella include visual dyslexia, auditory dyslexia, minimal brain damage, strephosymbolia, specific learning disability, word blindness, primary learning disability, cerebral dys-

function, neurological disorganization, and Gerstmann's syndrome, to mention a few.

Some of the experts choose to subdivide the etiology of "Dyslexia" under the headings of (1) congenital, (2) developmental lag, or (3) brain damage. It is highly improbable that heredity, late blooming, or physical accident could produce an identical problem or that the same remediation would be required in these very different situations.

Characteristics of "Dyslexia" are as varied as the terminology and the etiology. Some of the frequently listed characteristics include poor motor coordination, crossed dominance, reversals in letters and words, poor spatial orientation, poor auditory discrimination, confusion with vowel sounds, poor visual discrimination, poor memory for words, and hyperactivity.

Other "experts" have been known to state that the percent of "Dyslexics" varies from one tenth of one per cent to forty per cent. How could there possibly be such a range of probable occurrences? Obviously, this range could not exist if there were any kind of agreement as to what constitutes this ill-defined disability. The problem of "Dyslexia" is compounded because of lack of clarity. Since no one knows what it is or what causes it, how can anyone's definition

or etiology be wrong? As a result, any self-proclaimed expert can jump on the bandwagon and espouse his or her ideas, and this is precisely what has happened. On a recent television talkshow, a nutritionist stated that there is a forty per cent incidence of "Dyslexia." No statement was made to cite the source of the comment. So "Dyslexia" has in essence become a contagious disease and is becoming more prevalent as more and more ill-informed specialists, laymen, and parents join the parade. Some state legislatures have even passed laws concerning "Dyslexia." As a result even more parents will be bilked out of large sums of money by "Dyslexia" clinics. If the clinic gives a diagnosis of "Dyslexia," who can dispute it?

So much for the non-existent definition, characteristics and the opposing ideas of causation, let's look at some of the treatments.

Often the child is given more of the same thing at which he has failed, and hates with a passion, phonics. More of the same will probably increase the failure and create more distaste for reading.

In some cases the child may alternately be given pep pills and sedatives. Some of these medications are considered experimental and are sometimes dangerous. Some

1. DYSLEXIA – AN OVERVIEW

children spend time on a balance board or walking a balance beam, neither of which shows a relationship to reading, and sometimes tossing a bean bag is used in conjunction with the balancing.

There are various visual perception materials used for the "Dyslexic." Use of templates, tracing, connecting dots, following the swinging ball, drawing lines, working puzzles, and reproducing figures are often used to excess. These activities have some bearing on the development of a child in the quest for reading. However, in many cases the claims made by their advocates are unsubstantiated, and the overuse of the activities will bore the child. Research on visual training is contradictory, and many of the visual programs do not have much effect on reading per se.

One program suggests that the child has missed a step in development and must go back to the beginning to start over with creeping and crawling. This treatment becomes more ridiculous when it calls for complete avoidance of music. But that is not all. The child must also sleep in a particular position. Anyone can see that this program will most certainly improve reading!

Then there are some who believe eye-hand dominance to be at the root of the problem. If the child is right-eyed and left-handed, for example, the reading difficulty can be overcome by making the child right-eyed and right-handed or left-eyed and left-handed. Unfortunately for these theorists, there is little relationship between crossed dominance and success in reading. Directional confusion has a bearing on reading, but crossed dominance does not.

Many of the extremely poor studies which claim to show that the above-mentioned techniques are effective treatments for the "Dyslexic" were made by those who have a selfish interest in the technique be it prestige, financial profit, or otherwise. Also, the studies generally fail to take into account that correlation does not mean cause. The child may well have improved, not because of the particular treatment, but because something was being done. Quite likely improvement was a result of the individual attention which the child had not received prior to remediation.

At this point it is obvious that there is great confusion as to the causation, definition, terminology, characteristics, and treatment of "Dyslexia," despite the fact that much good research has been generated by university reading clinics. With this lack of agreement, it logically follows that there

should be no such term as "Dyslexia" and those who have the best interest of children in mind would perform a great service if they would stop pinning this meaningless label on children. Private reading clinics are notorious for this, although there are many which do not reap their profits by such scare tactics. The sure-fire cure for "Dyslexia" is to cease the usage of the term altogether.

The official position of the IRA prepared by the Disabled Reader Committee reads:

> There is no single cause for reading disabilities. Reading problems can be caused by a multiplicity of factors, all of which are probably interrelated. Just as there is no single etiology, there is no one choice of intervention. For those reasons we deplore the action of those individuals and institutions who suggest that their methods are infallible, appropriate and optimal for every child and universally efficacious.

Severe reading disabilities certainly do exist, but instead of mislabeling the child as "Dyslexic," the experts should find out the child's specific strengths and weaknesses. Then, based on the child's physical needs (visual, auditory, health), emotional needs, social needs, particular reading deficits, and preferred learning modalities the reading specialists, using an interdisciplinary approach, should plan a highly individualized program for the particular child.

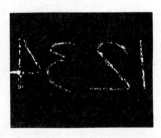

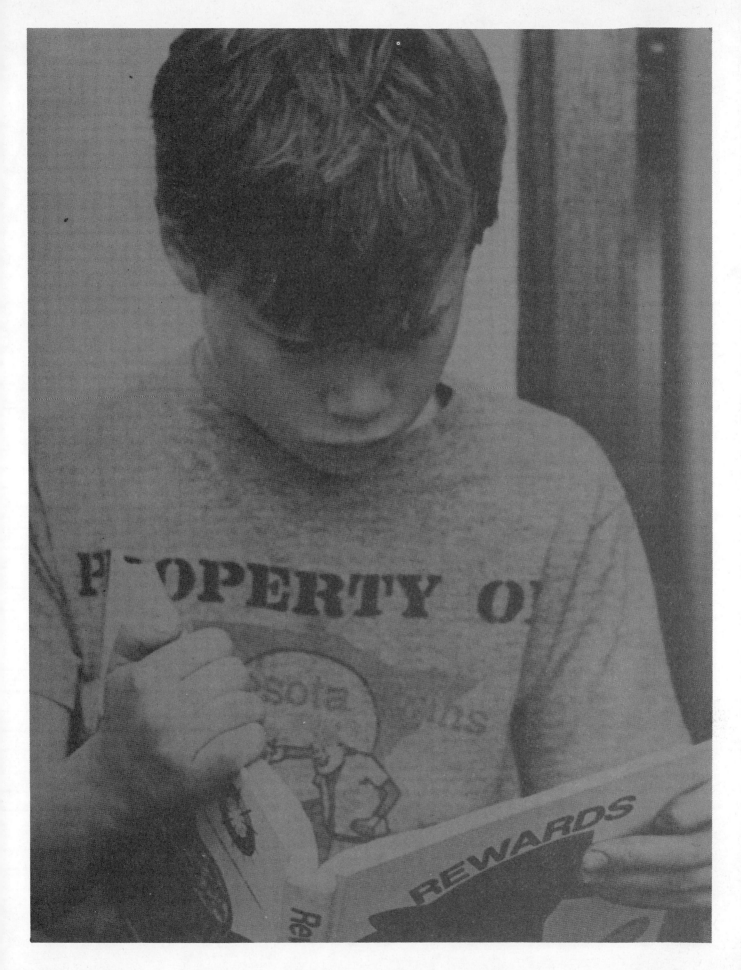

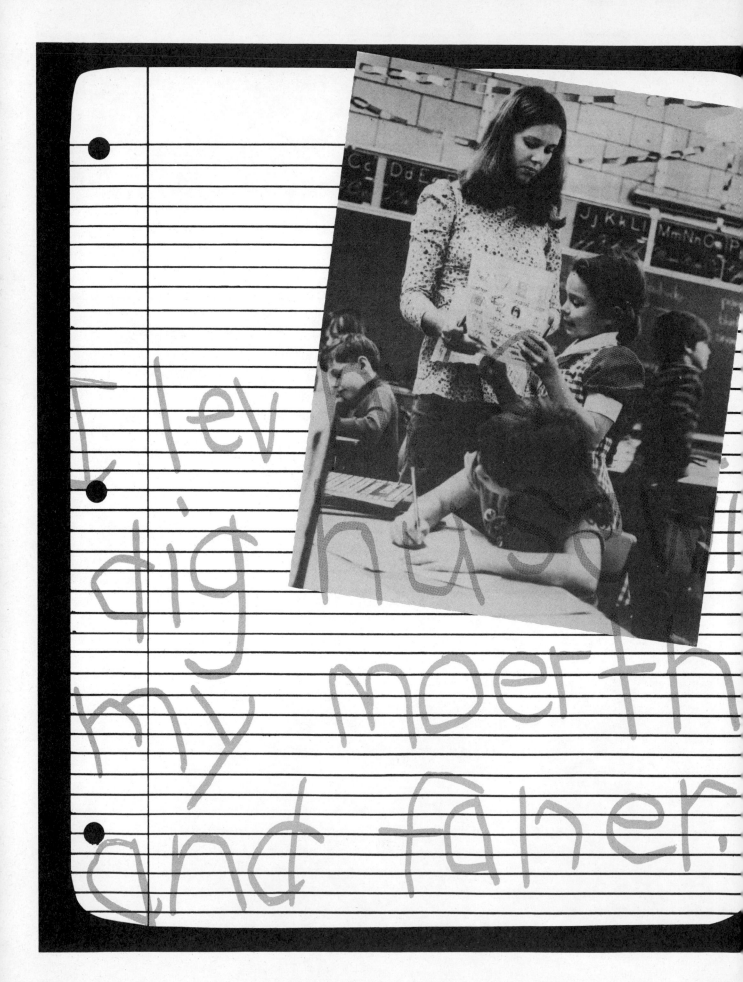

I lev
dig nusr
my moerth
and faher.

Diagnosis and Assessment

The process of diagnosing a reading disturbance serves as a manner of deriving instructionally relevant information for remediation. This is due largely to the close relationship between reading diagnosis and reading remediation.

The process of diagnosing a child's reading difficulties can be categorized into two basic approaches, informal techniques and standardized testing. Very often the classroom instructor may administer informal techinques, whereas standardized testing is normally conducted by specialized personnel.

One of the most crucial factors in informal assessment of dyslexia is close observation of the child's reading, both orally and silently. Particular aspects of the reading process must be considered for effective assessment. Some of these include the discerning of which word analysis skills the child utilizes, how extensive his sight vocabulary is, which consistent word analysis errors are made by the child, which particular words or parts of words are consistently distorted or omitted, and the speed of the child's reading. During the course of a school day, several opportunities arise to observe a child's reading ability. Through the use of a systematic recording of observations using anecdotal records or checklist, the teacher may informally assess the reading problem and devise a remedial program.

Informal diagnostic reading procedures may also include informal tests designed to provide information concerning specific reading skills. Because these objective tests usually measure skills which are directly related to classroom instruction, many are constructed by teachers themselves.

One further informal assessment technique is an informal reading inventory (IRI), a series of sequentially graded reading paragraphs taken from one source. This differs from a standardized reading test in that the child's level of competence is appraised without reference to other children.

The most traditional approach to reading diagnosis remains the formal standardized tests. The majority of diagnostic reading tests include subtests measuring word recognition, word analysis, comprehension, and other related components of general reading skills.

Certainly, the key to effectively improving a child's reading ability lies in the proper diagnosis of the difficulty. Through an appropriate assessment procedure, individualized remediation techniques will emerge. Only through carefully constructed programs based on each dyslexic child's individual difficulties, can successful reading improvement be realized fully.

RightNoW

Detecting Learning Problems Before Children Start School

—FRANKLYNN PETERSON
and JUDI R. KESSELMAN

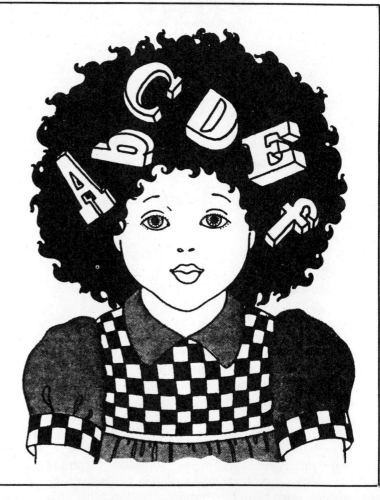

A statewide program in North Carolina helps insure that youngsters enter kindergarten both psychologically and physically prepared to learn. Three years ago, under the direction of psychologist Mary Haynes of the North Carolina Developmental Evaluation Centers, a network of 12 screening programs in which four-year-olds are given free comprehensive examinations were set up throughout the state. Trained examiners spot hidden problems that could hinder normal development or progress in school. Then they tell parents how to have those problems solved. They also pinpoint gifted children, so that parents and schools can provide adequately for them.

Dr. Haynes says, "About twenty-five percent of the youngsters have serious disorders that could handicap them in education or growth. Ten percent have vision defects, and eighteen percent have hearing loss. We detect hints of serious emotional disorders, learning disabilities and even incomplete immunizations."

Besides these problems, another 25 percent of the ex- amined children have correctable weaknesses that could slow them down in school. "We find weak pencil skills, poor language skills, poor eye-hand coordination and socialization problems," says Dr. Haynes. "Often they can be remedied."

Dr. Haynes believes that North Carolina's figures probably reflect the percentage of preschoolers all over the country who have undetected handicaps. She says, "The irony is kindergarten teachers used to complain that half their students began school with problems. We're finding they were right. But our job isn't just to diagnose; it's to correct the problems before the children start school by guiding their parents to the proper help."

Parents learn about North Carolina's Statewide Preschool Screening Program (SPSP) through TV, radio and newspaper ads, brochures in pediatricians' offices, letters from preschool centers and word-of-mouth. Children may be taken to one of the state's 12 centers for screening by appointment, but the program's screeners also go into nursery schools, Headstart programs and community centers. So far, about 20 percent of North Carolina's four-year-olds have been screened.

A reporter recently observed while one little girl was being tested at the Asheville center. Four-year-old Lauri was led into an office by screener Katrina Wilson. The two played various games involving matching pictures and then letters. Eventually Ms. Wil-

son held up a card printed with the word *NO*. Lauri incorrectly matched it with a card saying *OZ*. But she found the correct match for the next word, *EAT*. Ms. Wilson spent about an hour testing and evaluating the child's memory, perception, reasoning ability, balance, coordination, and so on.

In the meantime, Lauri's mother was being interviewed about her daughter's behavior at home and at nursery school. Afterward Ms. Wilson told her how Lauri's performance stacked up against that of other four-year-olds. Lauri, as is true with most children, came out above average in some skills, average in some and below average in others. Her mother was told about games she could play with Lauri that would help correct two of the child's weaknesses — pencil skills and hand-eye coordination. Mrs. Wilson made a note to follow up on Lauri's progress in two months.

How did Lauri's mother react to the exam? "You have no idea how good it is to have somebody assure you your child is normal!" she said.

If, in the preliminary screening, children are found

to have more problems than Lauri has, they are tested further by one or more of the center's specialists. (They include a psychologist, psychiatrist, pediatrician, physical therapist, social worker, educational psychologist, nurse and speech pathologist.) Since few children turn out to have only one problem, the eight professionals hold frequent case discussions. Then they refer the children to public or private counseling facilities, where payment is scaled to the family's income. If the staff has time, it treats low-income children at the center.

Several other communities have screening programs like North Carolina's, but nowhere is there another statewide effort. Illinois experimented with a similar plan, but ran into administration problems and dropped it, although the city of Evanston retained its program. A suburban St. Louis school district tests its preschoolers.

The large, western-based Kaiser-Permanente prepaid health organization routinely screens its subscribers' youngsters.

Unfortunately, the North Carolina screening program

may be limited to screening only a small percentage of preschoolers because of monetary reasons. But at least one child expert believes such an economy would be shortsighted. A pediatrician, psychiatrist and former director of HEW's Office of Child Development, Dr. John Meier, says, "Many of us tend to get our commitments backwards. We spend all that money on college when spending more on young children would bring the most long-term rewards. North Carolina has put together one of the most comprehensive programs I've ever seen. It not only informs parents but pursues them to insure that the uncovered problems are taken care of."

Dr. Meier would like to see programs like North Carolina's developed all over the country. "If a national network of screening centers had been funded after World War Two the average IQ in America today would be one hundred thirty instead of one hundred. We'd have very little illiteracy, fewer school dropouts, less juvenile delinquency. In general, we'd have a lot more happy adults."

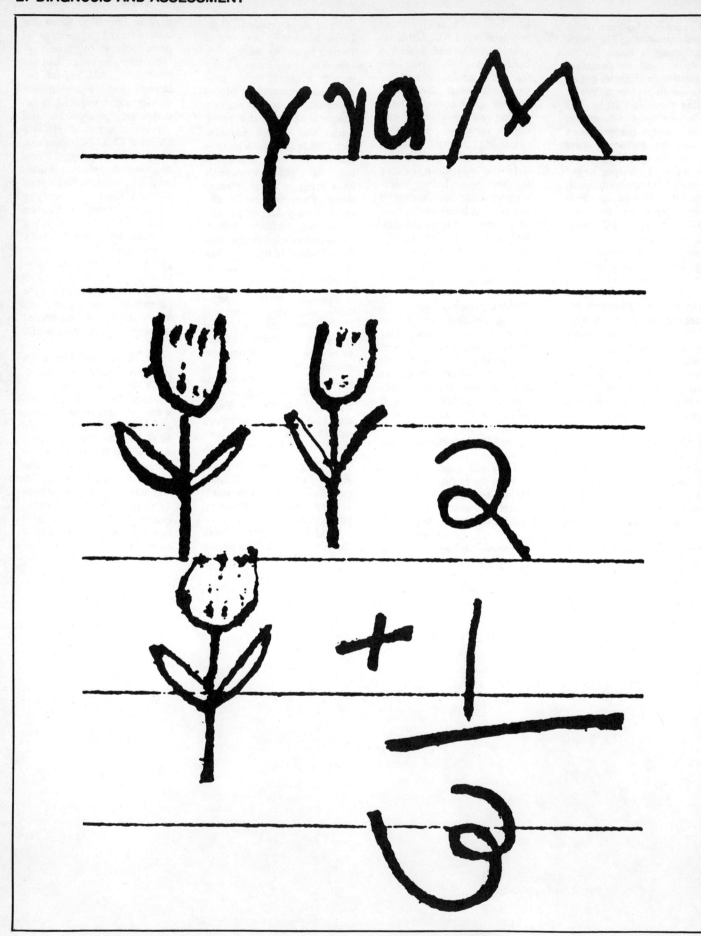

An Educator's Mystery: Where Do Performance Problems Come From?

Maxine Towle, PhD, and Allen Ginsberg

In this article pupil performance problems are examined as a function of environmental conditions in the classroom. Viewed in this light, the teacher becomes the key to the youngster's classroom success. To aid the teacher in taking the mystery out of performance problems, a process for performance analysis is presented.

When performance problems appear, disappear, and reappear as if under supernatural control, it is helpful to have either an exorcist or a set of powerful problem-solving tools immediately available. If requisitioning the services of the former seems absurd, then the only alternative is to utilize available scientific techniques for restoring appropriate performance. Available from the software of educational technology are two such techniques: task analysis and functional analysis. These two power tools increase problem-solving efficiency and when used consistently in the classroom, assist in the prevention of performance problems. This article will illustrate how these two power tools can take the mystery out of classroom performance problems.

THE TOOLS OF TASK ANALYSIS AND FUNCTIONAL ANALYSIS

Task analysis is the process of isolating, describing, and sequencing all the necessary subtasks which, when the child has mastered them, will enable him to perform the objective (Bateman 1971). This process tells the teacher what the child will have to know or be able to do to perform a given task. Assessing performance on the essential skills enables the teacher to pinpoint the missing skill. Individualized instructional programs may then be designed to teach the child.

Functional analysis is a diagnostic technique for identifying relationships between behavior and environmental events. Rooted in the history of scientific research, the procedure allows the user to be effective and efficient in identifying factors which are correlates of the difficulty. Crosson (1967) described a three-step analysis process functional for classroom use. The first step is to pinpoint the behavior in question, the second is to identify environmental conditions under which the pinpointed behavior occurs, and the third step is to identify those events which follow the occurrence of the behavior in question. The teacher implements the procedure by asking a series of questions:

(1) What is the exact behavior under question?
(2) How frequently does the behavior occur?
(3) What conditions precede the occurrence of the behavior?
(4) What events immediately follow the behavior?

Through this questioning process, the dynamics

"An Educator's Mystery: Where Do Performance Problems Come From?", Maxine Towle, Ph.D., Allen Ginsberg, *Journal of Learning Disabilities*, Vol. 8 No. 8, October 1975. ⁰1975 The Professional Press, Inc.

27

2. DIAGNOSIS AND ASSESSMENT

of classroom performance are described, and classroom events provoking and/or supporting the questionable behavior are identified. By analyzing performance in different settings and comparing the setting conditions, the teacher can isolate the events influencing the child's performance.

USING THESE TOOLS

A practicum student's (the junior author: AG) solution to a mysterious case of mirror writing illustrates the power of these two tools.

While thumbing through a pile of completed arithmetic worksheets, AG noticed an odd signature: Scrawled at the top of one of the papers was a conglomeration of letters that seemed to bear no resemblance to the name of any child in the class (see Fig. 1).

After a second examination of the signature, AG realized that this was Mary's paper. She had written her name as if she were looking in a

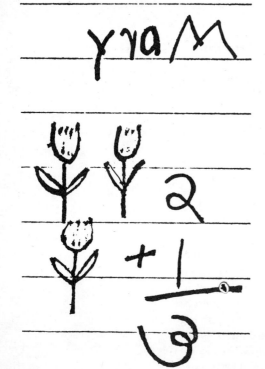

FIGURE 1.

mirror. He thought of the possibility of cerebral dysfunction and dyslexia, but knew that a premature diagnosis could prove damaging to Mary. More evidence of her mirrored writing would be necessary before any conclusion could be drawn.

AG then collected a sampling of Mary's school papers, and flipping through them he noted additional examples of reversed printing. There were arithmetic worksheets, vowel

exercises, and a variety of art projects in various stages of completion, all signed with either

YɿɒM or Mary

That afternoon AG confronted Mary with an example of each type of signature and asked if she was aware of any difference in the manner in which she had signed her name. She quickly labeled the mirrored one as being "backwards" and promptly corrected it. But a week later mirrored writing still appeared on some of her assignments.

The lack of consistency in Mary's performance was confusing, but at the same time suggested to AG the possibility that the problem had to do with the setting of the event rather than any internal dysfunction. He then decided to adopt a behavior approach toward Mary's problem. He hypothesized that Mary had learned somewhere along the way to print her name in reverse. Examining her papers for some sort of clue, he made an interesting discovery. Her mirrored signature appeared with the greatest frequency on art projects from the second half of the semester (Fig. 2).

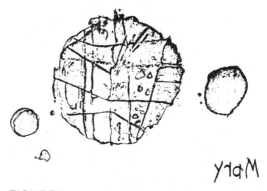

FIGURE 2.

Two days later he observed an art lesson. While he was waiting with anticipation for Mary to complete her drawings in order to see if his hunch was correct, the art teacher announced, "Only five minutes remain. Would everybody please clean up and remember to sign your name in the lower right-hand corner, just like real artists do." To illustrate her point she raised a piece of construction paper and indicated the lower right-hand area with a crayon.

Mary took her crayon in hand and carefully printed an "M" in the proper corner, and then paused for a moment, seeming undecided as where to place the "A." She finally settled on the left side of the "M," completing her name in the familiar, mirrored manner. Having identified the conditions of performance, AG mentally analyzed the requirements for task performance. Then, back in the classroom, he asked Mary once again whether she was aware of the way in which she had signed her art.

"You mean it's backwards," she replied. "I know, but it won't fit the other way." AG pointed out Mary's problem to the art teacher who in the next class changed the directions to "sign your name on the bottom of the paper." Mary then signed her name correctly. With this direction Mary was free to begin at any point and she elected to start far from the right-hand corner to allow room for all the letters in the proper sequence (see Fig. 3).

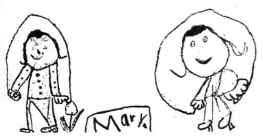

FIGURE 3.

THE POWER OF ANALYSIS

As shown in the case presented here, a problem in performance is the child's way of signaling a breakdown between task requirements and present skill level. When the teacher detects the signal, a task analysis will identify the performance component that is missing from the child's repertoire. Mary had already identified this component and was making compensation. AG's analysis of the task identified four basic skills for performance under the art teacher's command. In order to follow the teacher's directive, "Write your name in the lower right-hand corner," the basic skills required are: (1) to identify the lower right-hand corner; (2) to write the letters legibly; (3) to sequence the letters left to right; (4) to place the first letter far enough left of the right edge of the paper to allow space for all of the letters.

Spatial organization is an important skill in writing, but it is apparent only under certain directives. When conditions changed, as did the teacher's directions from the regular classroom to art class, the performance became susceptible to error because Mary had not been taught techniques of spatial organization in writing, such as starting at a hand's width from the corner of the page. This incident shows that during the early stages of skill development,

performance is highly sensitive to task directives. Unless all necessary subskills of performance are taught, dependency on specific performance conditions will be prolonged and the opportunity for deviance will be increased. However, if tasks are analyzed carefully prior to giving directions, performance will not become a mystery. Performance requirements will be identified before task demands are made and performance problems will not mysteriously appear.

Even with the best of intentions, problems may appear. For this reason it is also important that educators have tools to systematically study environmental/behavioral relationships in the classroom. AG had the powerful tool of functional analysis at his command. This procedural tool enabled him to efficiently identify relationships between classroom setting events and performance by pinpointing the processes which produce and maintain the behavior under question. Following the three-step process described above, AG first pinpointed the behavior in question, and then determined the occurrence of that behavior. The problem was "letters mirrored in signature." He identified the most frequent occurrence of mirrored letters as being in art projects.

He then identified the specific environmental conditions related to the differences in the frequency of deviant behavior by visiting the art class and noting the teacher's directions and Mary's performance there and in other curriculum areas.

The analysis was completed by the identification of events which supported or reinforced the deviant responses — events that happened immediately after the mirrored signature occurred. AG observed the teacher accepting Mary's paper and ignoring the mirror-written signature. Further, Mary was offered no help in learning to judge distance and so her mirror writing continued.

Following this procedure, AG was able to efficiently specify the relationship between classroom events and performance. It was clear that when given directions to write her name in the lower right-hand corner, Mary mirrored her name and no one corrected her. Since Mary could write her name correctly under other conditions, the art teacher agreed to change the directive. While this eliminated the problem, it was not completely corrected until Mary was taught how to judge the amount of space required for her name before starting to write.

Just how efficient was this procedure? AG, with one course in methodology and no previous practicum experience, solved the mystery

2. DIAGNOSIS AND ASSESSMENT

in under three hours after employing the technique of functional analysis. He not only helped Mary, but also increased the teacher's understanding that a child's performance may be highly sensitive to the task requirements as presented. Furthermore, this strategy made use of the available resources in Mary's educational program: the classroom teacher, the art teacher, and, most important, Mary herself. Needless to say, the child is often forgotten as being an available resource. Lindsley (1973) reminds us that the child knows best when we're talking about child behavior, and functional analysis emphasizes the importance of the child in understanding classroom dynamics.

DUAL TOOLS

Task analysis and functional analysis together are a strategic approach to solving performance problems regardless of the nature of the difficulty. The strategy involves both a logical and empirical process which can be used with the confidence that the results will be positive. As science has replaced magic, so the dual tools of task analysis and functional analysis have taken the mystery out of performance problems in the classroom — *Department of Studies in Behavioral Disabilities, University of Wisconsin, 2605 Marsh Lane, Madison, Wisc. 53706.*

REFERENCES

Bateman, B.: Essentials of Teaching: Dimensions in Early Learning Series. San Rafael, Calif.: Dimensions Publ. Co., 1971.

Crosson, J.E.: The functional analysis of behavior: A technology for special education practices. Ment. Retard., 1967, 7, 15-18.

Lindlsey, O.R.: Skinner to precision teaching. In J.B. Jordan (Ed.): Let's Try Doing Something Else Kind of Thing. Arlington, Va.: Council for Exceptional Children, 1973.

Genetic and Psychodynamic Aspects of Developmental Dyslexia— A Cybernetic Approach*

Hugh B. G. Thomas, M.A., D.P.M.

This paper sets out to provide a theoretical approach to cognitive functions and their acquisition, and includes discussion of brain damage, heredity, and family environment as factors in the genesis of dyslexia. The presence of "noise," not only in the brain itself, but also in the input data which it has to process, implies that inference *must play an important part in many psychological processes; language acquisition in particular appears to be one type of pattern-detection process involving inference. Whenever inferential procedures are used, standards of inference must be adopted. A method of estimating the standard (D) adopted by an individual on a given occasion, in a recognition-learning situation, is described and explained. If a child habitually adopted excessively lax or stringent standards in all matters or in specific areas of cognitive growth such as language or reading acquisition, this overconfident or overcautious attitude would have deleterious effects. It is shown that in 33 families attending a dyslexia clinic, a much higher proportion of the children than of their fathers or mothers had abnormally high or low D values by comparison with normal young adult students.*

Based on presentations given at the 5th and 6th Annual Workshops of the Dyslexia Memorial Institute, 1936 S. Michigan Avenue, Chicago, Illinois 60616.

In considering the possible effects of biological or psychological factors on the acquisition of a particular skill such as reading, the research worker or clinician of today has one great advantage over the 19th century neurologist. The development of the electronic computer has made it much easier to think clearly about questions such as the relationship between structure and function, or the "localization" of function in the central nervous system. When a program is read into a computer, it sets up a network of electrical pathways and these impose numerous constraints on the events which can take place when an item of input information is subsequently read in. To program a computer is to confer upon it a specific structure, or organization, which determines what its function will be. In short the content conferred upon the computer temporarily makes it into a working "machine."

Today this word need no longer conjure up the image of an oily, clanking engine. Anything which carries out a specific operation, characterized by certain constraints, is a machine. The word "noisy" is also defined more generally and no longer refers only to audible noise. A noisy machine, now, is one in which the constraints are not obeyed strictly but are blurred by arbitrary exceptions and violations.

2. DIAGNOSIS AND ASSESSMENT

It is not wholly "disciplined" but shows "initiative" (Turing, 1968). Most if not all biological systems can be formally described as noisy machines.

From this point of view, teaching a child to do arithmetic or to read is essentially a matter of building up the necessary "machinery" in his brain, while providing an emotional environment in which this slow process of organizational growth can take place properly. Emotional factors can interact with physical factors, such as brain damage or a limited biological potential for intelligence, so as to stop or restart the growth of a complex psychological skill or the growth of the personality in certain directions.

The presence of noise, not only in the functioning of the machinery itself but also in the data on which it has to operate, means that in order to discover the constraints which make various aspects of his environment to some extent predictable and manageable, a child must adopt methods of inferential reasoning broadly analogous to those used by statisticians. This in turn implies that *standards* of inference must be adopted and suggests that the adoption of unduly lax or stringent standards would have far-reaching effects on personality growth and cognitive development, including language and reading acquisition. In what follows, these arguments will be developed, a new method of estimating an individual's standards of inference will be described, and some results, obtained from children with reading problems and their parents, will be reported.

INFERENCE AND LANGUAGE

There are two ways in which a deficiency in some specific skill, or group of skills, might possibly be inherited. First, if specific genes could control the development of specific cortical areas, the inheritance of a faulty "regional gene" could no doubt cause the corresponding area to develop abnormally. However, it does not follow that the acquisition of information-processing functions normally conducted in that area would be affected. Unless the areas were very large or uniquely specialized, the situation would be equivalent to that produced by local brain damage in infancy, and the necessary machinery would presumably be set up in another area nearby. An alternative possibility is that if the specifications for setting up certain machines are conveyed as genetic information, a faulty specification could be transmitted in the same way.

If in fact some form of linguistic machinery is inherited, it clearly is not a ready-made language-recoding apparatus, fully capable of translating ideas and feelings into language and vice-versa. It must rather be a program for *learning* to recode: one which operates on examples of language experienced by the child in a variety of situations, in such a way that after interacting for some time with speakers of a particular language the child will have acquired "secondary" machinery for handling that language. The question of how this "primary program" (learning) works and what it does is central to the study of language and disorders of language acquisition.

Now it is a simple fact of observation that language is not random, but structured; a given word or phrase will occur frequently in some contexts and situations, but rarely or never in others. At the same time, it is known that this is no accident: a speaker or writer must choose, construct and order his words more or less correctly, not randomly, if he wishes to be understood. He must conform more or less strictly to certain social conventions which permit some sequences of speech sounds, symbols, words, phrases or sentences, but forbid others, if his language is to be meaningful to other people; others, for their part, must share substantially the same constraints — they must know the same language if they are to extract meaning from it. In complying with these *linguistic* constraints the speaker or writer necessarily produces sequences of language units which are *statistically* constrained — i.e., nonrandom and precise. In fact the generation of language, like that of any other organized behavior, can be regarded as a matter of subjecting what is originally random, unstructured activity ("primary noise") to the appropriate constraints (Thomas, 1969).

It is convenient to classify linguistic constraints into various types. For example, in any given language certain sequences of symbols and sounds are acceptable as words and others are not; some ways of modifying and combining words are permissible but not others; and so on. These comprise the "syntactic" constraints of the language. Other ("semantic") constraints have to do with the *content* of what is said — its logicality, or its factual accuracy.

Neither children nor adults always impose the appropriate contextual constraints on their language. Accepted conventions of realism, logic, grammar, and proper spelling or pronunciation are often broken, with the result that language becomes a less reliable vehicle for the communication of meaning — partially meaningless "nonsense" language is produced. If the constraints of word formation and syntax are too loosely imposed, language becomes ambiguous and vague; if logical "content" constraints are violated, it becomes inconsistent and self-contradictory; and a relaxation of reality constraints results in a form of nonfactual but otherwise perfectly intelligible language which one might call "fantasy." Again, the appropriateness — and the probability — of using one word or phrase rather than another in a given verbal context is normally very much influenced by the topic and also by the objective toward which the discourse as a whole is aimed. If these long-range constraints are not imposed, the discourse will be directionless and wandering. Similarly, in the case of dialogue, each speaker's choice of words is normally constrained to some extent by what the other speaker has just said; and if these constraints are lacking, the dialogue, regarded as a single discourse generated jointly by both speakers, will be incoherent and partially meaningless to a bystander.

These examples serve to illustrate the point that language is experienced as meaningful because, and to the extent that, it is produced not haphazardly but in accordance with many constraints which are shared by the recipient. These are manifested as contextual effects, owing to the fact that language is made up of words or other units which occur one by one in serial order. The nature of verbal language implies that memory must play an important part in both the generation and the comprehension of speech or writing. Clearly, if a speaker or writer is not to "wander" he must be able to remember what his topic or objective is; but memory is also required for the imposition of short-range constraints. It is very common for one part of a sentence to qualify, refer to, or agree with another part which may be separated from it by a number of intervening words or phrases. A speaker therefore must often have to plan ahead, or to remember and "look back at" the beginning of a sentence while uttering the end of it. Conversely a listener must be able to hold a more or less lengthy span of language units in some accessible form of serial storage if he is to understand speech, for the meaning of a phrase or sentence depends both on the words it contains and on their order. The same of course applies to reading (Thomas & Huff, 1971).

If the language units constituting an "ordered string," such as a sentence, could not all be held simultaneously in serial storage; or if they could not be *read out* from this store, preserving their serial order, an element of uncertainty would enter into the recognition of the string as a whole. This would now become a matter of weighing probabilities and making decisions on the basis of incomplete information — i.e., of inferential judgment.*

Next, it must be emphasized that the constraints of a natural language are not perfectly systematic and "regular" in the way that the rules of a formal language such as algebra are. They are not so much rules as *generalizations*, to which there may be a good many exceptions; and these, no less than the *rules*, must be observed when the occasion calls for it. This is why school children find themselves learning lists of irregular verbs, or nouns which violate the gender rules, and so on, when studying a second language. Nevertheless the generalizations still provide a valuable way of dealing economically with many individual linguistic facts.

This element of irregularity, or arbitrariness, has its origins in the long evolutionary history of the language. The concern here, however, is that it is present, not only in whatever second language the child may be taught at school but also in the first language he ever acquires. In this case the child usually discovers most of the generalizations for himself. Parents rarely give their infants formal lessons in grammar. They usually provide innumerable examples of more or less correct ordinary usage and correct a variable proportion of the child's mistakes. No matter how literate or conscientious the parents may be, because of the arbitrariness of the language (even in its purest form) the child will always be compelled to generalize on the basis of partially inconsistent data. Here again, therefore, some form of inductive inference must be involved.

The quasi rules which are the constraints of the language will usually have to be picked out from a confusing background of contrary

---

*As will appear later, inference is not a purely logical activity; factors such as "confidence" and "caution" enter into it. Consequently a short serial memory span (as in a child, or in someone dealing with a language in which he is not fluent) leaves more room for emotional considerations to affect the hearer's or the reader's interpretation of precisely what is said, which in turn affects his interpretation of what is meant. Did Elizabeth I of England say, "I have never said that I would marry anyone," or, "I have said that I would never marry anyone?" Which did her foreign suitors' envoys believe her to have said? And what conclusions did they draw, as to her intentions?

examples and exceptions. For example, a child may notice on a number of occasions that the plural of a certain kind of noun is formed by adding -es; perhaps his mother speaks of "a box," but of "two boxes"; of "one match" but "several matches"; and so on. The child, wanting one day to form the plural of "mouse," may well say "some mouses" — a rather common error, which presumably arises because the child has inferred that the -es rule is general for all nouns ending with sounds like "ks," "ch" or "ss" which are sibilant. When the mistake is corrected, the child learns that "mouse" is an exception; but the exceptions will not always conveniently occur after the child has formulated his generalization. Another child might encounter the word "mice" much earlier in his experience with plural nouns. It is rather as if the child were required to recognize a number of designs, all embedded in a network of added lines and some overlapping with others, except that the "designs" are not known to the child beforehand, so that he has to discover them for the first time and not merely to recognize them. In effect the acquisition of linguistic constraints is a form of *pattern detection* task in which regularities have to be discerned against a background of "noise." This type of problem arises very frequently in many different departments of everyday life for adults as well as children and for lower animals as well as humans. Almost every aspect of the physical and social environment is to some extent lawful, orderly, and constrained; but in nature as well as in language, regularity and order are almost always masked to some extent by arbitrary accidents and exceptions. Living organisms are constantly faced with the need to take advantage of any invariant, regular characteristics which their environment may possess (Ashby, 1956); and because these constraints are generally obscured by noise, their identification can only be achieved by what amounts to a process of inductive inference — i.e., of formulating hypotheses and modifying them from time to time in the light of fresh data.

Every child may thus be regarded as a kind of experimental investigator, continually trying to find out how things and people behave — that is, to discover the constraints which govern their responses to various kinds of event and incoming message. The acquisition of language, a progressive inferring of the rules together with a learning of the exceptions, then falls into place as one among many lines of inquiry which the child pursues at various stages of his development. At the same time as the child is discovering the principles of word and sentence construction, he is also beginning to find out the laws which govern (more or less strictly) many other aspects of his physical and social environment, and acquiring the means of imposing reality constraints on his language. Similarly, by listening to adults and interacting with them the child gradually discovers the rules which people obey (not always rigorously) when they argue and so develops the ability to impose logical constraints on his own utterances.

The acquisition of a nonverbal language, to be used mainly for the conscious or unconscious communication of emotional states, may be viewed in a similar way. So also may the development of personality, at least to the extent that the constraints which govern an individual's interpersonal transactions are determined by his construct system — i.e., by the system of hypotheses in terms of which he interprets the world, including himself (Kelly, 1955; Bannister & Mair, 1968). In short there emerges a picture of the child continually inventing hypotheses about the physical, human and linguistic environment in order to account for his observations; carrying out increasingly specific "experiments," both verbal and nonverbal, in order to check and refine his hypotheses; and using those hypotheses as a basis on which to *predict* other people, animals, inanimate objects and so on, for the purpose of either cooperating with them or controlling them.

HEREDITY, ENVIRONMENT AND DYSLEXIA

It seems therefore that some form of machinery for inductive inference is necessary for the acquisition and comprehension of language. A distinction is often drawn between verbal and nonverbal intelligence, but this does not necessarily mean that a special inferential machine is required for language acquisition as distinct from other kinds of inferential data processing. The differences may arise from the special nature of the data which must be processed, in the case of language acquisition. Again, supposing for the moment that a single, all-purpose inferential *program* is inherited, it does not necessarily follow that the infant's cortex contains only one inferential *machine*, which operates on all types of data. The original genetic specification could well be used to program several, perhaps many such machines, which would all operate in the same manner but on different types of data and in different cortical areas. A simple variant of this view would be that the neuroanatomical structure of, say, the entire "associative cortex" is genetically determined in such a way that the cells in any particular locality will operate inferentially on whatever input information may be routed to that locality.

Whether there is assumed to be one inferential machine or many, a defect in the genetic program would be expected to have a more or less drastic effect, from birth onwards, not only on the acquisition of language but in all aspects of cognitive development and personality growth except for those which call for little or no inferential thinking. But in order to account for a selective impairment of reading acquisition, it would be necessary to postulate additional genetic factors which applied specifically to reading — i.e., the visual as distinct from the auditory interpretation of language — or else to suppose that environmental factors, acting at the relevant time, could interfere with this particular aspect of cognitive growth. Indeed, the foregoing arguments might still apply even if the defect in the inferential program were not inherited but acquired in early infancy. In principle there are two ways in which this might happen. If this type of reasoning were normally taught to the baby, presumably by example, faulty teaching might produce a defective program. Alternatively, supposing that a faultless program were inherited, the development of secondary machinery for processing environmental data might still be delayed if the infant were exposed to an excessively noisy input from the beginning — e.g., if a mother's responses to her baby were highly capricious and unpredictable.

A number of investigators, avoiding the complex problem of how the hereditary transmission might be achieved, have tried to determine empirically whether the familial incidence of dyslexia does in fact conform to one or the other of the standard Mendelian modes of inheritance. These studies do not agree on all points and it is by no means proved that a single dominant gene is involved (Lenneberg, 1964). In fact it has not yet been strictly shown that the tendency for dyslexia to run in families is even partly due to genetic rather than psychological causes. To prove this it would at least be necessary to show that the incidence of dyslexia in identical twins of dyslexic parents is greater than in the same-sexed fraternal twins of dyslexic parents. Also, before any genetic study can be undertaken it is necessary to choose appropriate criteria for identifying the character which is assumed to be inherited. Genetic studies of dyslexia, however, have generally relied on tests of reading performance — i.e., tests which evaluate the functioning of the *secondary machinery* for reading. The state of development of this machinery at any given age must depend partly on the kind of input the child has received (Davis, 1947), and this would obscure the influence of a genetic factor specific for reading if one did exist.

It is difficult therefore to estimate the importance of heredity in the causation of dyslexia. However, Mittler (1969) gave the Illinois Test of Psycholinguistic Abilities (ITPA) to a number of 4-year-old twins and singletons, not selected on clinical grounds, and estimated that only about half of the variability of the test scores as a whole could be attributed to genetic variation. Since it is not known what specific psychological processes are required for the performance of the various ITPA subtests, the interpretation of this estimate is somewhat uncertain; but in the circumstances it seems fully justified to base both treatment and research on the assumption that psychodynamic factors within the family play a considerable part in the causation of dyslexia. This certainly does not mean that the parents of dyslexic children, any more than those of autistic children, should be made into scapegoats (Schopler, 1969). Even if they were solely responsible, for one to approach them in a spirit of moral condemnation would do more harm than good. On the other hand, it would be most unfortunate for the child if relevant emotional issues were ignored as a result of placing too much emphasis on any specific or nonspecific contribution which heredity or brain damage may make.

STANDARDS OF INFERENCE AND PSYCHOLOGICAL MATURATION

In formal research work, just as in the informal "research" of the growing child, the need for inferential reasoning arises from the fact that the relevant aspects of the data are obscured by noise. But what is relevant information and what is noise depends entirely on the nature of the inference in question. For example, suppose an investigator wishes to test the hypothesis that men are in general taller than women. (It will be assumed here that this hypothesis is in fact correct.) He will measure a sample of the general population and compare the mean heights of the men and the women, using the *t*-statistic (Weatherburn, 1962) or some other statistical measure of the "discriminability" of the two subgroups. His hypothesis dictates that

2. DIAGNOSIS AND ASSESSMENT

the observations must be classified according to sex; and the object of calculating t, say, is to determine whether or not a convincingly sharp distinction exists between the two sets of measurements so produced. This distinction would be absolutely sharp if sex were the only factor affecting an individual's height, but in reality it is only one of many. The others, which blur the distinction, are therefore sources of *noise* in relation to this particular hypothesis.

A more complex hypothesis, which took some of these other factors into account as well as sex, would enable the individual height measurements to be classified into a greater number of categories with less overlap between one category and another — hence fewer exceptions. Conversely, if the investigator chose to test an *incorrect* hypothesis initially and divided his sample on the basis of some factor totally unconnected with height, the two sets of measurements would not be statistically distinguishable. In short, a complex hypothesis yields a less noisy system of data classification than a ·simple one, so long as the increased complexity is due to the addition of valid assumptions. This argument applies equally to psychological hypotheses such as those involved in language acquisition and the growth of an individual's construct system. It implies, among other things, that an excessively simple language, such as pidgin English (Jespersen 1922), or an unduly simple conceptual viewpoint will add to the barrier of noise which to some extent isolates every individual from his social and physical environment. Both of these factors must apply in the case of the very young child and presumably a gradual noise reduction normally occurs, as the child gains a mastery of language and acquires an increasingly refined, complex but realistic construct system.

Returning to the original example, the calculation of t is a step in the procedure of testing the null hypothesis. It is an indirect method of determining the probability that a distinction as sharp as the one observed would occur purely as a result of noise, under the given sampling conditions. If this probability is found to be smaller than some criterion value P, the null hypothesis is said to be rejected at the significance level, or confidence level P. The investigator can then claim that the results require some explanation other than chance and that his hypothesis provides an explanation.

Within certain limits the choice of the criterion P is left to the investigator's judgment.

The more stringent the standard of statistical proof he means to adopt on a particular occasion the smaller the value of P he must choose. A P-value of 0.50 for example would be useless because a rejection of the null hypothesis by this criterion would leave a 50:50 risk that it was in fact true. However the choice of a more stringent criterion means, in general, that more data and more time will be needed to reject the null hypothesis in a case where it is, in fact, false. It is conventionally accepted that P-values below 0.001 are needlessly stringent for all normal purposes, whereas values above 0.05 are unacceptably lax. In other words, *according to the accepted convention among statisticians*, there is rarely so much at stake that a rejection of the null hypothesis at the 0.001 level cannot be taken as a certainty, or so little at stake that a rejection which fails to reach the 0.05 level can be regarded as valid.

Clearly, if inference plays a part in many of the information processing operations the brain is called upon to perform, then very often something must occur which is equivalent to the setting of a confidence level or some comparable standard. This conclusion opens up the possibility that for some people, the adoption of relatively lax or stringent standards of inference may be a more or less permanent individual characteristic — as if one investgator were always content to move on to the next step of his research after proving his current hypothesis only at the 0.05 level of confidence; whereas another might insist on testing every hypothesis at the 0.001 level.

Carried to the extreme, either tendency would clearly be maladaptive and pathological. An individual who was always satisfied with, say, the 0.20 level of confidence would be mistakenly rejecting null hypotheses, or accepting the less valid or two alternative hypotheses, about one fifth of the time. Consequently he would often try to explain facts which required no other explanation than chance or coincidence. He would tend to jump to conclusions — i.e., to be convinced too quickly on too little evidence. He would show poor judgment in choosing the most likely interpretation of the facts and would be uncritically accepting of facile explanations and conjectures. In short one might describe him as "gullible" or "suggestible" and his approach to hypothesis testing as "overconfident." Clinically he would probably be said to have a deficiency of "reality testing" and a tendency to "premature closure." He might also be said to show a "delusional" style of thinking but his delusional beliefs, though held with conviction at any given time, would be readily changeable rather than fixed in their content. One thinks of the excessively compliant, perhaps delinquent or "hysterical" individual with a somewhat formless personality and a vague or labile construct system, easily led and perhaps easy to hypnotize.

At the other extreme someone who habitually sought to achieve the 0.00001 level of confidence, for example, would be excessively anxious not to fall into these errors. He would rarely be wrong, but would be interminably slow in reaching decisions or in committing himself, genuinely, to opinions. Once having done so, after much hesitation, he might well be inflexible and obstinately resistant to changing them. Here one thinks of the detached, uncommitted person with an overriding need to be always right; hairsplitting, hypercritical, mistrustful of new ideas and often of those who propound them, but capable of achieving work of high quality if he happens to possess the drive required to come within reach of his own standards. His rejection of all but the most rigorously tested hypotheses might well cause such a person to develop a "blinkered" view of the world which would cater for some dimensions of experience with great sharpness and clarity, while leaving others vague or leaving them wholly out of account.

With regard to the child's acquisition of the spoken or written language, the view that this depends heavily on inductive inference is gaining ground among psycholinguists (Ingram, 1968) and it implies that there is a strong resemblance between language acquisition and tasks of the concept formation type studied by Bruner, Goodnow and Austin (1956). These authors noted that their subjects seemed to vary greatly in the criteria by which they decided, either that they had discovered the correct hypothesis, or that they should continue to ask for more data. It is a reasonable assumption that differences of a similar kind, perhaps even more marked than in the case of adults, would exist between one child and another. Aside from any influence heredity may exert, it is easy to see that a wide variety of psychological circumstances might cause a child to adopt overconfident or underconfident (lax or stringent) standards of inference, either in all matters or else in some specific area of experience such as the acquisition, recognition and interpretation of language.

A child who applied excessively strict standards, when acquiring the constraints to be obeyed in recoding spoken language into "meanings" and vice-versa (within the limitations imposed by a still-developing construct system) would be expected to make abnormally slow progress in learning to talk, like the investigator whose research is delayed because he aims ·at excessively high standards of statistical proof. Such a child might appear to know more than he believed himself to know. Conversely a child with unduly lax standards might make rapid progress but gain only a superficial and inaccurate grasp of the language, as a slipshod investigator does of his subject. The same arguments would apply to reading, at a later stage. The child must now acquire two more codes, two more sets of constraints: those which will relate the written language to meanings on the one hand and to the spoken language on the other.

METHOD

The following task was used originally to investigate the psychopathology of severely, acutely disturbed young adults and their parents (Thomas et al., 1971), but experience has shown that it can be given without alteration to children as early as the eighth year of life. It requires the subject to learn a target list of 15 numbers drawn from the range 0-99. The target list is presented at least five times and after each occasion the subject's knowledge of it is tested by a recognition method. This consists in presenting 100 numbers drawn from the same range, one at a time; the subject must decide whether or not each of these test numbers was in the target list and mark a check or cross in the appropriate place on a special response sheet, taking care to omit no responses and to make no extra responses.

Each target number occurs just once in the course of a given test series but the subject is not informed of this fact. The various test series are all different and the target numbers occur in a different random order, randomly placed in the sequence in each case. However, the test series is carefully designed to meet certain statistical criteria of similarity, randomness and uniform representation of the numerical range 0-99. The numbers are prerecorded on tape and the target numbers are presented at a fixed rate (one per 3 seconds). The test numbers are played back one by one as the subject indicates he is ready. Subjects are instructed to go at their own speed and are given no inducement to hurry, but in practice they very often set as fast a pace as the tape allows and in that case the numbers are presented uninterruptedly, at regular 3-second intervals.

Two measures of performance are computed

for each test series from the frequencies of correct and incorrect affirmative responses. These measures are derived from a statistical model of the main psychological processes involved in recognition memory, which was developed from a "decision-making" hypothesis of the processes involved in the detection of stimuli in the presence of noise (Tanner and Swets, 1954; Tanner, 1956; Parks, 1966). The underlying assumptions have been extensively tested and the fact that it has been difficult to distinguish experimentally between different variants of the model (Lockhart and Murdock, 1970; Banks, 1970) means that for practical purposes it may not matter greatly which version is used to interpret the test data.

According to the assumptions of the model as applied to recognition *learning* (Thomas and Patel, 1972), one performance measure (d') reflects the degree of statistical discrimination achieved during a given test series, by a process which compares each test number with the contents of a store containing a more or less unreliable, imperfectly learned and noisy version of the target list. It is assumed that the "recognition strength" signals produced by this process are subjected to an inferential decision-making procedure, equivalent to choosing one of two alternative hypotheses, which determines whether each signal is sufficiently strong to justify an affirmative response, or not. It is also assumed that during each test series, this decision process is biased in such a way as to yield the maximum possible satisfaction to the subject. This assumption makes it unnecessary to know what payoffs the subject awards himself for correct and incorrect affirmative or negative responses during any given test series. The second measure (v), which can never exceed 1 by definition, can then be interpreted as showing how closely the subject's performance at any stage approaches that level which would satisfy him completely.

The great majority of normal adults, children over eight years, and even severely disturbed psychiatric patients obey a "law" connecting v and d' so that, subject to certain precautions, it is possible to estimate statistically the value of d' at which v would equal 1 for the individual in question; that is, the degree of discrimination between target and nontarget numbers which he would accept as "perfect" during the course of learning. This value (D) can therefore be regarded as a measure of the extent to which the individual sets himself perfectionistically strict standards of inference, or the opposite. It can also be interpreted as a t statistic with 101 degrees of

freedom, if certain additional assumptions are made. From this point of view a D value of about 3.40 would mean that the subject set himself a standard equivalent to the 0.001 level of confidence, whereas a D value of about 1.69 would correspond to the 0.05 level. A D value much above or below these limits would imply that the subject was adopting unduly stringent or lax standards *compared with those conventionally adopted in statistical work.*

During the development of this method D values were obtained for 37 ostensibly normal young adults, mainly students, with no history of psychiatric consultation or treatment. According to the test, one of these subjects was severely perfectionistic, with a D value of 7.88 which lay more than four standard deviations above the group mean. Treating him as an atypical "outlier," the mean D value for the remaining 36 subjects was 3.66 with an S.D. of 0.675. It follows that for subjects of this age and socioeducational class, assuming an approximately gaussian distribution, about 95 percent of D values should normally lie between 2.31 and 5.01, and about 99.7 percent between 1.64 and 5.69. In other words values outside these two ranges may be regarded as abnormal or exceptional at the 0.05 and 0.003 levels of significance respectively. It is noteworthy that the mean (3.66) corresponds to a standard roughly equivalent to the 0.001 level of significance.

Some insight into the psychological significance of a relatively high or low D value in normal young adults can be gained from the following result. Twenty of the subjects just mentioned, not including the outlier, completed the MMPI questionnaire within a few days of performing the recognition-learning task. Only one of the correlations between D and the subject's uncorrected T-scores on the 13 standard MMPI scales reached significance, namely that between D and the *Psychopathic Deviate (Pd)* score; this was negative ($r = -0.51$, $p < 0.05$) and almost reached the 0.02 level of significance. Evidently for this type of subject a relatively low D value tends to be associated with a pattern of MMPI responses which in young adults and teenagers is thought to be typical of the delinquent, risk-taking personality, whereas a high D value is associated with a low *Pd* score, which seems to be typical of the conventional, conforming individual with narrow interests (Dahlstrom and Welsh, 1960). The characteristics of normal young adults with relatively low and high D values therefore broadly agree with the predictions made earlier, concerning the kinds of personalities to be expected in individuals with overconfident and overcautious standards of inference.

Clinically, a considerable proportion of dyslexic children seem to fall into one or the other of these categories — at least in matters connected with reading; and as one aspect of a larger study, D values have been measured for an unselected series of children, all referred with reading difficulties, and for their parents, with the preliminary object of estimating the incidence of extreme D values in such families. No attempt will be made here to examine any relationships which may exist between the children's D values and other clinical or psychological test data, but it is relevant to mention that the children's ages ranged from 7 years 11 months to 15 years 6 months.

RESULTS

Out of 36 complete family triads seen during the period of this study, the father was not available to take the recognition-learning test in one case; in another, the father learned the target list very rapidly so that the correlation between v and d', though large, was based on too few test series to reach significance and his D value was therefore invalid; and in a third family the child (age 6 years 9 months) yielded an invalid D value because the correlation was too small to reach significance even with a relatively large number of test series. The table therefore refers to the 33 families in which the child, mother, and father all had valid D values, based on significant correlations ($p < 0.05$) between v and d'. Values below 1.64 or above 5.69, being also below 2.31 or above 5.01 respectively, are represented twice in the table, to show how the incidence of extreme D values

TABLE I. *Incidence of extreme D values in referred children and their parents.*

	D-VALUE				
	Below 1.64**	Below 2.31*	2.31- 5.01	Above 5.01*	Above 5.69**
Children	2	7	17	9	6
Mothers	2	3	29	1	0
Fathers	1	3	28	2	1

* Values more than 2 S.D. above or below young adult norm ($p < 0.05$)

** Values more than 3 S.D. above or below young adult norm ($p < 0.003$)

in these families compares with the distribution in normal young adults.

The striking feature of the results is that whereas relatively few of the parents' D values

are high or low , extreme values are common among the children. For example the three highest values (9.57, 9.54, and 9.17) were all for children. Half of the children had D values more than two standard deviations above or below the young adult norm of 3.66, whereas the proportion is much less than half for the mothers ($\chi^2 = 18.94$, $p < 0.001$), and for the fathers ($\chi^2 = 16.03$, $p < 0.001$).

DISCUSSION

There seems no reason to suppose that extremes of perfectionism or laxity in hypothesis testing would be confined to children with reading difficulties; rather it seems likely that disorders of inferential judgment — i.e., of "common sense," would give rise to a wide range of educational and behavioral problems and might well set the stage for serious difficulties in later life. Conversely, a variety of problems might be avoided or relieved if means could be found to prevent the overconfident or overcautious attitude from developing or to correct it. Apart from psychotherapy or medication, some form of adaptive teaching machine capable of giving immediate feedback based on repeated computations of the child's D value could well serve to give such children a "feel" for more appropriate standards of judgment.

However a number of questions remain to be answered by further research. Is this high incidence of extreme D values a feature only of disturbed children or will it also be found in problem-free children? The age factor may be important here; it may be, for example, that very young children tend in general to have more variable standards or a higher incidence of extreme standards, and that certain kinds of family influence are needed to establish stable standards in the normal range. The effects of varying the task itself also need to be explored. It is not necessarily the case that all types of subject would give similar D values on the present task and a visual analogue of it, or on a version which used concept acquisition in place of recognition learning. — *7B Oriel Road, Fulwood, Sheffield 10, Yorkshire, England.*

REFERENCES

Ashby, W. R.: *An Introduction to Cybernetics.* London: Chapman & Hall, 1956.

Banks, W. P.: Signal detection theory and human memory. *Psychol. Bull.,* 1970, 74, 81-99.

Bannister, D., and Mair, J. M. M.: *The Evaluation of Personal Constructs.* New York: Academic Press, 1968.

Bruner, J. S., Goodnow, J. J., and Austin, G. A.: *A Study of Thinking.* New York: John Wiley, 1956.

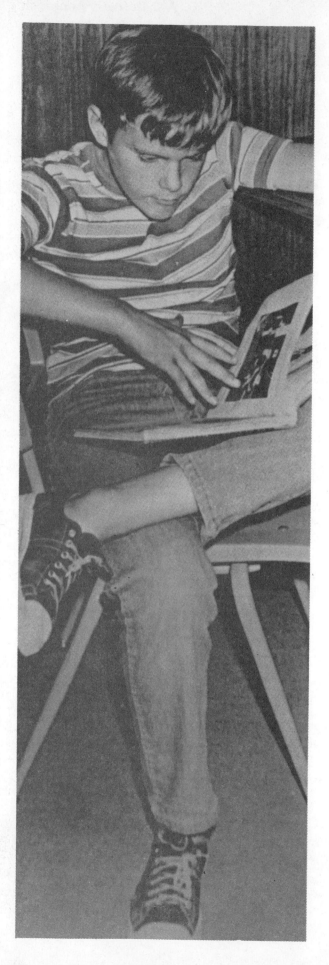

FOCUS

Two Perspectives Concerning Dyslexia:

Medical and Educational

The literature on the medical perspective first appeared in England with an article written by a physician (Morgan 1896). Since that time many other investigators have attempted to find medical explanations for poor reading or dyslexia, including Hinshelwood (1917), Schmidt (1918), Orton (1937), Hallgren (1950), Hermann (1961), Critchley (1964), Money (1966), and Johnson and Myklebust (1967). In the past seventy years, over 20,000 books, articles, and papers have been published on the subject; they have sought a common behavior pattern among all dyslexic children and clearcut evidence of a neurological etiology (Eichenwald 1967). The difficulty in finding empirical evidence to support the medical perspective is that it is almost impossible, even at present, to directly examine the brain of the child. Therefore, evidence of dyslexia owing to brain damage or dysfunction is most difficult to establish diagnostically and is necessarily presumptive in nature.

Educators, reading specialists, and psychologists generally have a different view of dyslexia from that of the medically oriented scholars. The early studies of children who could not read (Monroe 1932, Robinson 1946) investigated the causes of reading failure, including the neurological factor; but these investigators concluded that the neurological theories of causation had not been strongly established. Vernon (1957) concluded that the term dyslexia was unacceptable because the condition is not comparable to alexia. Bond and Tinker (1967) also maintained that it is impossible to distinguish dyslexia from a severe reading disability and that "the clinical worker may question the value of the term."

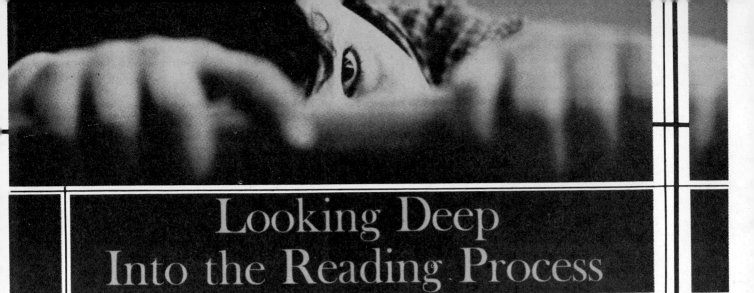

Looking Deep Into the Reading Process

Implications of the two perspectives of dyslexia.

What are some of the implications of the differences in these two perspectives? For purposes of discussion the two frameworks will be called the *medical perspective* and the *educational perspective*.

> 1. While the scholars working within the medical perspective search for a single etiological factor as causal, the scholars in the educational perspective seek a combination of causes, stressing that it is not likely that a single factor can be shown to be causal.

> 2. The educators are likely to place greater emphasis on the developmental sequence of reading skills, making an intensive search for the child's break with the developmental reading pattern. The medically oriented investigator is likely to place greater emphasis on the language-related areas, such as speech and oral language skills, as well as on other related disabilities, such as arithmetic skills, perception, motor development, and social skills.

> 3. For the educator, alexia, or the loss of reading skill in the case of an adult, is different from the inability to learn to read in the case of a child. Therefore, the term dyslexia is not generally used among this group. They emphasize the necessity of differentiating "maturational lag" from central nervous system dysfunction.

> 4. Educators see the diagnosis of dyslexia as lacking operationality in that it does not lead to appropriate teaching strategies. After the diagnosis of dyslexia is made, one must still investigate what reading skills are lacking, how the child best learns, what are the appropriate materials to overcome the problem, and so on. The diagnosis of dyslexia alone provides few clues as to the appropriate treatment and remedial measures.

> 5. While the medically oriented clinician is likely to focus solely on the disabled child and to emphasize individual treatment, the educator is likely to perceive a broader role and function within the school and to devote a portion of his time and energy to the developmental reading program of the entire school in seeking preventive measures.

In conclusion, there are two strands of thinking concerning dyslexia that have been developed by two separate fields of study: (a) the medical perspective, and (b) the educational perspective. The review of the literature on dyslexia does not lead to conclusive evidence for or against the approach of either discipline. Each researcher and scholar must and should study the reading problem of children in terms of his own training, experience, and framework. Each discipline has built a substantial body of literature, but neither is benefiting sufficiently from the work and foundation that has already been made by the other. If children who cannot read are to be helped, disciplines must forget labels and begin to work together.

The National Advisory Committee on Dyslexia and Related Reading Disorders was created by the Secretary of Health, Education and Welfare in 1968 to investigate, clarify, and resolve the controversial issues surrounding dyslexia. The Committee report, released by HEW in August 1969, reported the following information about dyslexia: "In view of these divergencies of opinion the Committee believes that the use of the term 'dyslexia' serves no useful purpose" (National Advisory Committee on Dyslexia and Related Reading Disorders 1969, p. 38). Perhaps more important, however, the Report recommended to the Secretary of the Department of HEW several vital steps to improve the reading of students within our nation who experience difficulty in learning to read.

One of the key recommendations was the creation of an Office of Reading Disorders within an appropriate agency of the Department of Health, Education, and Welfare.

"I Can Think, But What's Wrong is My Words

Dyslexia

WHEN A CHILD IS PRESENTING PROBLEMS OF BEHAVIOR OR PHYSICAL SYMPTOMOLOGY, INCLUDE THE LANGUAGE LEARNING DIMENSION IN ASSESSMENT OF CAUSE AND PLANNING OF DESIRABLE TREATMENT

Margaret B. Rawson

Mrs. Rawson is Editor of the professional journal in this special educational field, *Bulletin of the Orton Society*, and is a language consultant. She has been active in the field of remedial reading since the 1930's.

The title for this article on dyslexia was suggested by the elaborated chief complaint of 10-year-old Alfred. The following could be his own self-descriptive statement:

"What's wrong is my words. It always has been. It makes me mad, because I can understand and I can think. It's just the words. When I was very little they said I didn't seem to hear folks talk, although I heard the bell ring and the dog bark — but I soon caught on. I knew what Mom and Dad were saying, but I got my own sounds tangled up and couldn't say what I wanted to. Sometimes I couldn't think of the right words. Sometimes I still can't, but now I can think of others, and after a while the just right ones sometimes pop up.

"About the biggest trouble with me is that I forget the words I want to read. Either I just can't learn them, or I work very hard and do learn them, only I forget them right away, or some I know so I mostly get them right but without warning they get away. Then the other kids say I'm dumb, and I know the teacher and my folks think so, too, whatever *they* say. I guess I am, because I know I work hard, even though the grown-ups say I'm lazy. You should hear my teacher. She gets mad when I forget. She says, 'You know that word. You knew it yesterday. You could read it if you'd only try!' But I can't help it. I *do* try, but I forget, even if only some of the time.

"I have a hard time with writing and spelling, too. I can't seem to make the words look right. That is harder than reading them, because I have to think them up in my own mind and make them just right, no guessing. Make one letter wrong and you're done! I know why they say, 'Mind your *p's* and *q's*.' I'm always getting them backwards; *b's* and *d's*, too, and lots of others, and when I mean to write *saw* it's just as likely to come out *was*, or *left* may get to be *felt*. Lots of times they don't even look like real words, they are so twisted up.

"Then there is the trouble with what I write — but nobody else can read it. I can't read it myself, to tell the truth. It doesn't look the way I mean it to, my hand gets all tightened up and tired. It's slow, too. People are always saying, 'Do hurry up! You're keeping us all waiting.' I feel like a dummy. I get so fed up I have to go to my shop and make something — and then do I catch it for not doing homework!

"My big brother used to have trouble, too, but he can read now. He still can't spell, though, and he gets bad marks on his work because of that in high school. My older sister stutters like nobody's business. Dad says my little brother 'is all thumbs

"'I Can Think, But What's Wrong Is My Words,'–Dyslexia," Margaret B. Rawson, *Medical Insight*, December 1970. •1970 Insight Publishing Company.

and has two left feet!' My baby sister (she's four) — well just try to understand her! But to hear them talk about my two other sisters, well, they just whizzed through school and college, and everybody asks, 'Why can't you be bright like that?'

"My dad says to cheer up, though, because he was dumb in school and hated it — but look at him now. Maybe he can't tell left from right, but he has a good job with high pay, and he says I'll probably be able to make a living, too. Actually, we have a lot of mixed up lefties in our family, like my mom and Uncle Jim, but I can use one hand about as well as the other, one for some things and the other for others. I tell you, we're a crazy, mixed up family, all right!

"They gave me some tests the other day and the man says I'm bright but that I've got real problems. He can say that again! I heard the man who gave the tests tell Mom it was 'a bad case of *dyslexia*' or something like that. It sounded so awful Mom cried. He said we could do something about it if we just get the right teacher, one who can teach me the way I can learn. All I have to say is *let's hurry*, because this word business is driving me crazy. I'm either going off my head or I'm going to get mad and smash things up."

Many young patients who come to the attention of the physician, be he general practitioner, pediatrician, ophthalmologist, psychiatrist or otologist, are somewhat like Alfred. They are usually referred for some other reason — vague stomach complaints or vomiting in the morning on school days. This may be because they are withdrawn or erratic or disruptive, or with such statements as, "If he can't read, there must be something wrong with his eyes," or, "Maybe it's his hearing — could be that's why he can't speak clearly and doesn't pay attention." Perhaps, his elders think, it is anxiety or tension or his way of getting attention.

Layman and professional alike, we all tend to fit any strange phenomenon into our familiar frames of reference. Life is such a complicated affair that it is rare that any patient will not have at least some symptoms or circumstances to which one could attribute school failure. If, however, further inquiry reveals learning problems like Alfred's, even though the child "seems bright" and there are no physical findings to account for his failure, it is quite possible

that his is a case of dyslexia (*dys* — poor or inadequate, *lexia* — from *legein,* to speak, hence *lexis* — words, in their lexical sense).

This condition, since its first published descriptions, has been called by 40 or more names, some emphasizing symptomatology, some etiology, some social or educational problems, some indications for treatment, and some a mixture of these and other elements. First it was called congenital word-blindness by Drs. Hinshelwood, Morgan and Kerr, working independently in England in 1895 and 1896. While Hinshelwood later thought of these cases as probably more numerous in fact than on record, it remained for the American neuropathologist and psychiatrist, Dr. Samuel T. Orton, and his associates to demonstrate the prevalence of specific language disability or strephosymbolia (the twisted symbols of which Alfred is complaining). A now commonly used term is dyslexia, or more accurately developmental dyslexia. In 1968, nineteen members of the World Federation of Neurology's Research Group on Developmental Dyslexia were drawn together from four continents to discuss this world-wide problem. In a rare instance of international and professional unanimity, they came up with this definition for dyslexia: "A disorder in children, who, despite conventional classroom experience, fail to attain the language skills of reading, writing and spelling commensurate with their intellectual abilities." Having ruled out the things it was *not*, they agreed that this disorder "... is dependent upon fundamental cognitive disabilities which are frequently of constitutional origin."

We may look upon these children as being at the ineptitude end of the continuum of a capacity for learning human verbal language, which is the last skill acquired in human evolution — one requiring a most complex integration of cortical functions. Recent evidence from the laboratories of neurophysiology and neuropsychology tends to substantiate Orton's hypothesis, that this is a problem of neurophysiological variation, not a defect nor a disease. However, since many man-hours have been spent on the question of definition without universal agreement, perhaps it is better left at the level of Alfred's self-diagnosis, for it is here that we may be able to do something immediately helpful. "What's wrong is my words. I forget them — the look, sound and feel of them — even though the grown-ups say I am bright and have nothing else wrong with me, and I've had schooling that worked all right for the other kids."

How many of these children are there? Figures vary widely, because of differences in definition and standards of case selection. This is only part (but a

Dyslexia

**to fsih als
i liev ni a
huose wil
my faimly**

very significant part) of the nation's admittedly serious reading problem. **The dyslexia component of the problem is 10 percent of the otherwise normal population. These persons have sufficient disability to prevent them from attaining functional competence in school; another 10 percent is unable to achieve at or near their intellectual potential. Many of these young people are unrecognized or inadequately treated. But once the physician is aware of the syndrome, he is likely to find quite a few of them among his patients. There are at least four boys to each girl. Dyslexia occurs among the middle-class and well-to-do families as well as among those of lower socio-economic status, although the complications of poverty seem to exacerbate any condition. My own experience suggests that in our current justifiable concern for the disadvantaged, we may be overlooking the needs of the non-poor children, condemning them to failure or under-achievement, with personal and social consequences which are wasteful at best, and often disastrous.**

These results may be devastating for any child, in terms of frustration and loss of a sense of self-worth, especially during the school years, when achieving competence is the main business of psycho-social development. We see this in the disruption of school, home and neighborhood life, and in the high rate of school failure, dropout, delinquency, unemployability and neurotic disturbance among unhappy and frustrated non-readers. It is particularly striking in the relatively unproductive lives of those who "just get by", far below the levels of their potentialities.

Children may, and often do, have more than one handicap, be it physical, neurological, emotional, socio-economic or education. But when a child is presenting problems of behavior or physical symptomatology, it is helpful to include the language learning dimension in assessment of cause and planning of desirable treatment.
The doctor will be alerted by findings or history of:

► Early incomprehension of *speech*, delay in learning to talk, persistence of mis-articulation, distortion of sound-sequence in speech, difficulty in word-finding and self-expression, marked and persistent stuttering or cluttering;

► After school entrance, inadequate or erratic memory for *printed words,* reversal of orientation or sequencing in spatial patterns, with consequent misreading of words, lack of development of adequate word-attack skills in spite of some instruction (which, to be sure, is by no means universally to be counted upon);

► *Spelling* which ranges from the frequently unconventional to the bizarre, and is generally below the level of reading competence (which, in turn, is likely to be below achievement in arithmetic and other subjects insofar as they are not dependent on reading);

► *Penmanship* which may (or may not) be slow, poor in form, irregular in slant and general appearance and often not as the writer intends it to come out;

► A kind of *non-specific clumsiness* or perhaps motor difficulty shown only in the writing of letters and numbers while large and small muscle skills permit excellence in sports and in fine handwork such as model-building;

► Late *choice of handedness* and continued confusion or uncertainty about left and right, geographical directions and, in extreme cases, other dimensions, such as time and up-down, and the like;

► *Familial incidence* of any of the above symptoms, in variable patterns.

Emotional disturbance, whatever its manifestations, may be either concurrent or consequent upon the language problems, but is, our experience suggests, seldom specifically causal. When present, as it usually is, it serves to tangle the evidence and sometimes to complicate the treatment, although success in learning often obviates the necessity for specific treatment of the emotional problems.

A few simple tests in his office will take the examining physician a long way toward a tentative diagnosis of dyslexia and suggest further referrals to colleagues with special fields of competence in this respect. In this quick series of screening tests one might ask the child to: write his name; tell the date and his birthday; name the days of the week and tell which comes before Wednesday and after Thursday; point to his own left ear with his right hand and tell which is the left hand of the examiner who sits facing him; read a short paragraph which seems to the examiner "probably too easy" and then one or two progressively harder ones; write in his own spelling, "I am a big boy," and "This is my very best writing." If he is older, he might write a few sentences or a short paragraph to dictation and read a paragraph from a newspaper. Let him draw a bicycle, and hop across the room on one foot and back on the other. It is surprising how much the physician can thus find out about his young patient's language-related development in a very short time.

If dyslexia seems the likely verdict, a refinement of diagnosis is highly desirable before treatment is begun. Ideally, one refers the child to a language disorder clinic, but these are regrettably scarce. A clinical psychologist should be consulted if possible. The results of group psychological tests, such as those given in schools, are unreliable for these children, since they rely on the use of verbal, often reading, skills and on clerical facility which are just the handicaps in question and which therefore intervene between the child's true intelligence and its demonstration. An assortment of other exploratory tests of visual, auditory and motor skills and achievements can be drawn on as the experienced clinician thinks appropriate. Thus the specialist will substantiate and amplify the diagnosis and be able to advise the parents, either directly or through the physician, as to the appropriate educational treatment.

While there are more uncertainties and fewer justifiable pronouncements in this field than most, one can say with assurance that, "However the diagnosis is arrived at, the effective treatment of dyslexia depends on education." Appropriate remedial training administered individually, in a therapeutic climate by a skillful teacher with relevant special education and experience in this field, is the optimum answer. Some good work in early preventive programs with properly screened classes is now being done. Treatment of older children can sometimes be carried out satisfactorily in very small groups. However, students differ so widely that the efficiency of the instruction is likely to be less than in the situation in which teaching can be individually tailored to the initial and developing needs of the child.

The absolutely necessary condition for this sort of program, however, is the careful, continuous supervision by a highly qualified specialist-teacher. The remedial education of a dyslexic child is not a job for an amateur, no matter how kindly, well-meaning, or even skilled in some other form of teaching or helping. The chances of failure are too great, and *this* child cannot afford another failure or the time which would be largely wasted en route to such failure!

During the past 45 years, educational procedures have been refined which do make the successful education of most dyslexics possible. The best of these are closely tied to understanding of the neurophysiological and neuropsychological development of the human being, the structure of the language to be taught, and the individual patterns of strengths and relative weaknesses of each diagnosed individual. "Teach the language as it is to the child as he is," is the simplification often used. But the actual process, like the language and the child on whom it depends, is by no means simple. The underlying principles were formerly held to be uniquely appropriate to children with language disabilities, but are now beginning to be accepted as desirable in general curricula; for dyslexic children they are quite essential.

Since whole words are configurations too large and complicated for these youngsters to master and retain as units, they are broken down into their coded elements, the sounds of speech and the letters used to represent them. These are taught thoroughly, through all the appropriate sensory modalities — *visual, auditory* and *tactile-kinesthetic* — and continuously re-synthesized into words and sentences which carry meaning. This is a *structured, systematic, cumulative* and *thorough* building up of understanding and skill in the language forms of the mother tongue. The objective is to make them automatically useful in reception, formulation and expression of thought; but at the same time to build in a set of rescue-techniques, to be used in moments of unpredictable breakdown to which the dyslexic individual will always be more or less prone. These constitute a store of back-up knowledge, by the conscious use of which the dyslexic can think his way out of an *impasse.*

Being an expert in this field is truly a "large order." It points to another serious manpower shortage which must somehow be met if Commissioner of Education Allen's "Right to Read" objectives are to be reached by the millions of children who are likely to have the greatest difficulty in becoming fully literate.

What is the outlook for these children? Can boys like Alfred be helped to "make it" in an America built on a foundation of literacy? Alfred, of course, is a rather fictitiously articulate composite of the many boys and girls known to diagnosticians and teachers of dyslexic youngsters. However, given recognition of their problems and support in solving them, dyslexics *need not fail,* nor even lower their academic and vocational sights.

On a case basis there are many hundreds, even thousands, of young people who, in the past 45 years, have been helped back into the academic mainstream, or, identified early, have been so taught that they never left it. Unfortunately, not many of their stories have been published, either biographically or as contributions to statistical studies, but they do exist. Under even reasonably favorable circumstances, experience encourages us to say that a dyslexic student of any age, child or adult, can learn to read up to the level of his intelligence, to write legibly though perhaps not beautifully, and to spell well enough to hold his own until his wife and his secretary can take over.

Biographies of such illustrious men as Edison, Hans Christian Andersen, Harvey Cushing, Albert Einstein, Auguste Rodin, A. Lawrence Lowell, and many others, including perhaps the greatest of them all, Leonardo da Vinci, give evidence that their subjects struggled with some of the same problems which have plagued Alfred. Like many lesser folk they made some adaptation and went on with their careers. Many others, less able to cope with their difficulties, have joined the ranks of the quietly, or unquietly, desperate.

We cannot, in the present state of knowledge, prevent dyslexia, any more than we can prevent tone deafness or make tolerable musicians of everyone, but enough is known so that we can prevent many of the problems that stem from it. If we identify these individuals with variant learning patterns as early as we can, and often this is the physician's opportunity, and give them the right kinds of educational help, we can make a large contribution toward the solution of the problems of school failure, illiteracy, underachievement and the waste of one of our most valuable national resources — human potentiality.

SUGGESTED READING

1. Critchley, MacDonald, M.D.: The Dyslexic Child. London, Heineman, 1970. Springfield, Illinois. C. C. Thomas, Publishers.
2. Money, John, Editor: Reading Disability: Progress and Research Needs in Dyslexia. Baltimore, The Johns Hopkins Press, 1962.
3. Orton, Samuel T., M.D.: Reading, Writing and Speech. Problems in Children. New York, W. W. Norton, 1937.
4. Rawson, Margaret B.: Developmental Language Disability: Adult Accomplishments of Dyslexic Boys. Baltimore, The Johns Hopkins Press, 1968.
5. Thompson, Lloyd J., M.D.: Reading Disabiltiy: Developmental Dyslexia. Springfield, Illinois. C. C. Thomas, 1966.

Reversals in Reading: Diagnosis and Remediation

SANDRA B. MOYER
PHYLLIS L. NEWCOMER

Abstract: Traditionally, a great deal of significance has been assigned to reversal errors in reading and writing. These errors are commonly attributed to perceptual difficulties that reflect neurological immaturity or deficiency. This article takes the position that reversals are not caused by perceptual defects but often result from the child's inexperience with directionality as a salient feature in making discriminations, and with proper instruction, even 4 and 5 year olds can learn to distinguish between reversible letters. This view is supported by a review of relevant research. Guidelines for diagnosis and instruction are presented.

SANDRA B. MOYER *is Lecturer, Division of Education, College of Multidisciplinary Studies, The University of Texas at San Antonio; and* PHYLLIS L. NEWCOMER *is Assistant Professor, Beaver College, Glenside, Pennsylvania.*

FOR many years, the tendency of many children to reverse letters or words when they write or read has received a great amount of attention in education. Although this behavior is recognized as normal in 5 or 6 year old children and is expected to disappear without special attention during the first or second grade, it causes concern when it persists beyond that time. When this occurs, these errors, termed *reversals*, often are regarded as an indication of perceptual disorders resulting from neurological anomaly or developmental delay. They are considered by many specialists in reading and learning disabilities to be symptomatic of a serious reading problem, sometimes referred to as dyslexia. Indeed, so much significance has been attributed to reversal errors that educators and other professionals such as neurologists, optometrists, and ophthalmologists have developed various remedial programs to correct them. Many of these programs provide the basis for special education interventions with the so called perceptually handicapped child.

The assumption that reversal errors reflect perceptual deficits has serious implications for the children who exhibit such errors. Clearly, these assumptions should not be maintained without substantial evidence supporting their validity. This article presents the view that much of the ominous significance attached to reversal errors is inappropriate. The authors take the position that first, the prevalent assumption that reversals are caused by perceptual disorders that reflect impaired neurological processes or developmental deficits is erroneous, and second, reversals often result from nothing more than a child's unfamiliarity with the concept of directionality as it relates to letter discrimination. The authors' opinions are supported with conclusions drawn from a review of the relevant research and the implications of their positions for teachers are discussed.

A Perceptual Deficit

Currently the term *reversal* is used to denote several distinct types of reading errors. Confusion between letters that are mirror images of each other, such as *b-d, p-q,* and, less frequently, *m-w, u-n,* and *t-f,* is one type. Reversal of short words, such as *on-no* and *was-saw,* is a second type. A third type involves only the reversal of certain letters within a word, such as *from-form.* Finally, changes in word order within a sentence are occasionally considered to be a type of reversal error.

Quite often, children who make any of these reversal errors are described as seeing things backward or as having mirror vision. This designation implies that the child actually perceives the image of the letter or word as it would appear in a mirror (e.g., *b* reflects as *d*). Actually, even if this explanation of reversal errors were accurate, it can apply logically to only the first type of error, confusion between letters such as *b-d,* since these pairs of letters have the same form and vary only in their position in space (i.e., their orientation). In other words, *b* and *d* are shaped identically and are differentiated only by the direction of the loop; consequently, they are mirror images of each other.

Such is not the case with the other three types of reversal errors. Word pairs such as *on-no* or *was-saw* do not form mirror images, a fact that can be easily verified by printing these words on a card and holding it up to a mirror. It would be even more difficult to explain reversals in letter order within a word and in word order within a sentence as seeing backward. It seems unlikely that a child would see only some letters or words backward and not others. It does seem plausible to assume that the latter three types of reversals are not errors in letter orientation or direction but are more accurately classified as errors in letter sequence. Liberman, Shankweiler, Orlando, Harris, and Berti (1971) provided some support for this conclusion. They found that among second and third grade poor readers reversals of letter orientation such as *b-d* and reversals of letter order such as *was-saw* were not covariant but constituted two distinct categories of reading errors.

In this article, the authors are particularly interested in those reversals that may be attributed logically to perceptual distortions resulting in seeing backward (i.e., errors in letter orientation). Although they account for a small percentage of reading errors—10% according to Liberman and others (1971)—they provide the foundation for many commonly accepted theories regarding the causes of reading disability.

The most popular and influential theory regarding the causes of orientation reversals incorporates the concept of cerebral dominance that was proposed originally by Orton in 1925. He used the term *strephosymbolia* or twisted symbols to describe errors of this sort and considered them to be an important cause of reading disabilities. According to Orton, reversal errors were due to a conflict between mirror image representations of a symbol in the right and left hemispheres of the brain. When neither hemisphere was dominant, the two conflicting mirror images created perceptual confusion. Reversal errors, therefore, were indicative of perceptual disturbance caused by a neurological malfunction.

Currently Orton's conceptualizations regarding cerebral dominance have little credibility among neurologists. The concept of hemispheric dominance has been supplemented in modern neurological theory by the concept of hemispheric specialization—the idea that each hemisphere performs certain functions more efficiently than the other. Recent evidence suggests that some of these functional differences between the hemispheres, and certain anatomical differences as well, are present quite early in life (Wada, 1974; Entus, 1975). In addition, there has never been any substantiation for the notion that mirror images are projected onto the brain, and many theorists regard this conjecture as illogical. For instance, Corballis (1974) has noted that one might as well expect the right and left sides of a camera lens to project mirrored versions of a single image. In short, there is no apparent reason for educators to accept this theory as an accurate explanation of reversals.

Despite these objections, Orton's cerebral dominance theory is the basis of the most popular maturational explanation of reversal errors that assumes young children lack a dominant cerebral hemisphere and must reach a certain level of maturity before developing a fixed lateral dominance. Children who lag in this development are said to lack the perceptual organization that is necessary to recognize the correct orientation of letters. Consequently, they make reversals. This mmaturity, termed mixed dominance, is also demonstrated by an inability to establish a dominant hand, foot, and/or eye.

The assumption that letter reversals are related to confused lateral dominance is accepted as fact by many educators although its veracity has never been established empirically. The interested reader is referred to a discussion of this topic by Shankweiler and Liberman (1972). Perhaps the persistence of the conviction that a causal relationship exists between the development of lateral dominance and reversals is due in part to research studies that suggest children's reversal errors are related to their level of maturation and they decrease as children get older. For instance, Davidson (1935) concluded that left-right reversals of the letters b-d and p-q were confused by more than 90% of kindergarten children and that it was not until the age of 7½ years that 50% of the children were able to perform this task without error. Jordan (1973) found that the incidence of left-right letter reversals dropped sharply between the ages of 6 and 7½ years. Gibson, Gibson, Pick, and Osser (1962) found that reversals constituted approximately 45% of all errors for 4 year olds, dropped sharply to about 23% of all errors for 5 year olds, and fell to about 5% by the age of 7. These and other such studies have been interpreted as supporting the notion that reversals occur because children have not yet developed the level of perceptual maturation that is necessary to perform the task.

The critical point in interpreting the results of studies of this sort is that they measure only how children typically behave and do not address the causes of children's behavior. What appears to be a clear maturational pattern may in fact reflect children's opportunities for learning a particular kind of right-left or up-down discrimination. Young children may have lacked the opportunity to learn these skills. As Hendrickson and Muehl (1962) pointed out, "Age norms derived from tests built to assess a given skill level provide no certain evidence as to what age they might first be taught and learned provided the learning conditions were effectively arranged" (p. 238).

A Learned Cognitive Skill

Actually there is considerable evidence that maturational level does not affect reversal errors. If the ability to detect differences in letter orientation depends upon the child's having reached a certain level of maturation,

as is often concluded from the studies cited previously, then attempts to teach this skill to children who are younger than age 6 should be unsuccessful. In fact, the experimental evidence is to the contrary. A substantial number of studies, which have been represented in Table 1, show that even 4 and 5 year old children can be taught to discriminate between mirror image forms when the nature of the discrimination is clear to them. These studies indicate that the ability to detect letter orientation such as left-right and up-down relationships among 4 and 5 year olds is primarily a learned cognitive behavior, not a developmental perceptual skill.

In examining the research under consideration, two factors emerge that seem to be necessary to assure that young children will be able to make mirror image discriminations. First, it must be clear to them that the orientation or direction of letters is the basis for the same/different judgment. In other words, children's attention must be drawn to the directional differences between the symbols. Since orientation as a distinguishing feature may represent a new concept, the children may have to be reminded often that it is relevant to the discrimination they are trying to make.

Second, the ability to discriminate between mirror image forms must not be made more difficult by a memory requirement, particularly in the beginning of training. The forms to be learned should be presented simultaneously so the difference between them can be examined. For example, the letter b should be presented with d and their directional differences emphasized (Samuels, 1973).

Some of the research studies listed in Table 1 suggest methods by which the directional aspect of mirror image forms can be brought to children's attention. In the Jeffrey (1958) study, 4 year olds were taught to push a button on the left or right that corresponded to a raised right or left arm on otherwise identical stick figures. After learning to grasp the right or left orientations, the children were able to learn to name the figures successfully. Hendrickson and Muehl (1962) taught a group of 5 year olds to match an arrow pointing in the direction of the letters b and d. The children were subsequently able to demonstrate that they had mastered the discrimination. Caldwell and Hall (1969) used transparent overlays printed with one orientation of a nonsense form (geometric shapes) as a sample and had children match this to other orienta-

TABLE 1

Representative Studies Investigating Discrimination of Mirror Image Forms by Young Children

Study	Year	Age of subjects		N	Description of Results
		Mean	Range		
Jeffrey	1958	4-4	3-11 to 4-9	28	13 of 14 subjects given motor response training learned to correctly label (Jack or Jill) identical stick figures with right or left arms raised.
Hendrickson and Muehl	1962	5-11	5-1 to 6-11	49	90%[a] correct responses by two experimental groups in matching the letters *b* and *d* to pictures following discrimination training (30 trials).
Wohlwill and Wiener	1964	Not reported	3-11 to 4-8	24	80% correct response for discrimination between left-right orientation of nonsense forms.
Over and Over	1967a	4-1 6-0	3-6 to 4-5 5-6 to 6-5	48	75%[a] of the 4 year olds and 100% of the 6 year olds reached criterion on discrimination of mirror-image oblique lines (/ \).
Over and Over	1967b	6-1	5-6 to 6-5	16	94%[a] subjects reached criterion (4 successive correct in 40 trials) in same/different judgment of kinesthetic differentiation of mirror image obliques.
Caldwell and Hall	1969	Not reported	5 to 6[a] yrs.	72	65%[a] subjects successful in a same/different pencil and paper task similar to the Davidson (1935) study after training designed to focus attention on orientation as a criterion for simultaneous matching.
Bryant	1969	5-3	Not reported	24	95%[a] correct responses (8 trials) in discrimination of oblique mirror image forms in a simultaneous presentation.
Cairns and Steward	1970	Not reported	4-2 to 4-10 5-2 to 5-10 6-2 to 6-10	60	30%[a] of the 4 year olds and 85% of the 5 year olds made fewer than 3 errors in discrimination between vertical and lateral reversals of the letters *A, T, U, B, D,* and *E.* The 6 year olds made almost no errors.
Koenigsberg	1973	4-11	4-1 to 6-0	120	Stimuli were filled triangles in different orientations and the letters *b, d, p,* and *q.* It was found that having the children focus on a demonstration by the examiner was as effective as a sensorimotor training technique in teaching discrimination of orientation.
Samuels	1973	Not reported	5 to 6 yrs.[a]	90	80%[a] of the subjects were successful in naming the letters *b, d, p,* and *q* following discrimination training.
Bryant	1973	4-7	4-5 to 4-11	160	The mean error rate for discrimination of mirror image obliques in simultaneous presentation was 2/20 for 4 year olds and 5/20 for 5 year olds.
Harris, Le Tendre, and Bishop	1974	5-1	4-10 to 5-4	18	95%[a] correct discrimination (8 trials) of mirror image obliques with no straight lines (e.g., card edge, table top) in the visual field to provide a source of reference.

Note: Socioeconomic status of the subjects, where reported, was middle to upper middle class.

[a]Approximate.

tions of the same form. Only when the child could match the forms without rotating the sample were the two figures judged to be alike. In this way, the directional aspect of the forms was emphasized and the children were able to learn to match on this basis. Koenigsberg (1973) found it equally effective to have the examiner demonstrate and explain the directional differences between geometric shapes and the letters b, d, p, and q.

Conclusions

The results of the research reviewed above suggest that for the most part children's confusion of mirror image letters is not caused by perceptual deficits but relates to the fact that they are unfamiliar with this type of discrimination task. The ability to successfully discriminate between such letters can be learned easily by most children before first grade when they are instructed properly. Until children encounter those letters of the alphabet that have mirror image counterparts, they have no occasion to consider spatial orientation when identifying objects in the environment. A chair is recognized and called a chair no matter which way it faces. In fact, the ability to ignore the position of an object in space is the basis for acquiring object constancy. It is a skill that develops early in life. McGurk (1972) has demonstrated that infants as young as 6 months are capable of recognizing abstract forms as identical in spite of different spatial orientations.

It would seem that the optical characteristics, that is, the purely visual impression of mirror image forms, are distinct. For example, b and d look different. It is possible, however, that for young children the spatial orientation that differentiates b from d is not a significant feature for identifying or naming things. The child must learn the importance of this particular feature. In any event, regardless of the probable causes of letter orientation errors, children can learn to make these distinctions.

Implications

This fact presents several implications for educators. For one thing, when children have difficulty with reversible letters, teachers may assume it is probably not due to developmental immaturity, undeveloped lateral dominance, or perceptual deficits that reflect neurological impairment. Rather, they should consider that such children may not have learned the importance of directionality as a distinguishing feature. By accepting this premise, reversals are appropriately regarded as relatively trivial and easily corrected errors, not as indicators of internal pathology or serious reading problems that must be remediated with special perceptual training materials. The most beneficial teacher response to such errors is to plan a suitable instructional program for the child. The following guidelines are provided to aid such instructional programing.

1. The discrimination task should be taught early, preferably as children are beginning to learn the alphabet. Delayed instruction of this concept may make it more difficult for children to learn reversible letters since they will be confronted with additional tasks such as learning letter names.

2. Instruction should begin with a simultaneous matching-to-sample task. For example, the child should select from among b, d, p, and q the letter that matches in orientation a sample letter b while the sample is available for comparison. This procedure serves to focus attention on the direction of the letter as the critical distinctive feature. The teacher may emphasize the directional differences between the letters by pointing them out and explaining them to the child. For some children, the use of motor activities such as having the child point in the direction a letter faces or using overlays like those employed in the Caldwell and Hall (1969) study may be useful for assuring attention to the relevant features of the letters.

3. When the direct matching task has been mastered, the teacher should present a delayed matching task. In direct matching, the sample letter is available for comparison; in the delayed task, the child must remember the orientation of the letter while looking for a match. To do this successfully, the subject must remember the direction the letter is facing rather than rely on direct comparison. There is some evidence (Harris, Le Tendre, & Bishop, 1974) that using the same letter for several consecutive trials facilitates this type of learning.

4. When memory for the direction of the letters is accurate and automatic, the child should be taught the letter names (Samuels, 1973).

5. In the instances where the teacher encoun-

ters an older child who exhibits confusion of letter orientation, the preceding guidelines may be used in somewhat reverse order to determine the source of the problem. For example, when a child reads the word *dig* as *big*, the teacher should ask the child to first say the letters in the word. If this is done accurately and the word can be reread correctly, the child's error was probably due to haste or inattention. If the child continues to name the letter incorrectly, the next step is to determine whether a simultaneous matching task can be performed. When given the letter *b* as a sample, the child must be able to choose the *b*'s from an assortment of *b*'s and *d*'s. If the child is successful in this step, the teacher must see if the letters that match the sample can be found after it has been removed from view. In other words, the child must remember the orientation of the letter. If this can be done consistently, the teacher may assume the problem lies with confusion of the letter names and a careful reteaching of these must be initiated.

In the unusual instance where an older child cannot perform the simultaneous matching task correctly, training programs such as those suggested in the first step of the instructional guidelines should be used to focus attention on orientation of the letters as the distinguishing feature. Should a thorough training program of this type fail, the teacher might then be justified in considering the possibility of a perceptual or neurological problem and might refer the child to appropriate specialists for further evaluation and treatment.

References

Bryant, P. E. Perception and memory of the orientation of visually-presented lines by children. *Nature*, 1969, 224, 1331-1332.

Bryant, P. E. Discrimination of mirror images by young children. *Journal of Comparative and Physiological Psychology*, 1973, 82, 415-425.

Cairns, N. U., & Steward, M. S. Young children's orientation of letters as a function of axis or symmetry and stimulus alignment. *Child Development*, 1970, 41, 993-1002.

Caldwell, E. C., & Hall, V. C. The influence of concept training on letter discrimination. *Child Development*, 1969, 40, 63-71.

Corballis, M. C. The left-right problem in psychology. *The Canadian Psychologist*, 1974, 15, 16-33.

Davidson, H. A study of the confusing letters b, d, p and q. *Journal of Genetic Psychology*, 1935, 47, 458-468.

Entus, A. K. Hemispheric asymmetry in processing of dichotically presented speech and nonspeech sounds by infants. *Biennial Meetings of the Society for Research in Child Development*, April 1975, Denver, Colorado (Abstract)

Gibson, E. J., Gibson, J. J., Pick, A. D., & Osser, H. A developmental study of the discrimination of letter-like forms. *Journal of Comparative and Physiological Psychology*, 1962, 55, 897-906.

Harris, P. L., Le Tendre, J. B., & Bishop, A. The young child's discrimination of obliques. *Perception*, 1974, 3, 261-265.

Hendrickson, S. N., & Muehl, S. The effect of attention and motor response pretraining on learning to discriminate b and d in kindergarten children. *Journal of Educational Psychology*, 1962, 53, 236-241.

Jeffrey, W. E. Variables in early discrimination learning: 1. Motor responses in the training of a left-right discrimination. *Child Development*, 1958, 29, 269-275.

Jordan, B. *The Jordan left-right reversal test*. San Rafael CA: Academic Therapy Publications, 1973.

Koenigsberg, R. S. An evaluation of visual versus sensorimotor methods for improving orientation discrimination of letter reversals by pre-school children. *Child Development*, 1973, 44, 764-769.

Liberman, I. Y., Shankweiler, D., Orlando, C., Harris, K. S., & Berti, F. B. Letter confusions and reversals of sequence in the beginning reader: Implications for Orton's theory of developmental dyslexia. *Cortex*, 1971, 7, 127-142.

McGurk, H. Infant discrimination of orientation. *Journal of Experimental Child Psychology*, 1972, 14, 151-164.

Orton, S. T. "Word-blindness" in school children. *Archives of Neurology and Psychiatry*, 1925, 14, 581-615.

Over, R., & Over, J. Detection and recognition of mirror-image obliques by young children. *Journal of Comparative and Physiological Psychology*, 1967, 64, 467-470. a

Over, R. & Over, J. Kinesthetic judgements of the direction of line by young children. *Quarterly Journal of Experimental Psychology*, 1967, 19, 337-340. b

Samuels, S. J. Effect of distinctive feature training on paired-associate learning. *Journal of Educational Psychology*, 1973, 64, 164-170.

Shankweiler, D., & Liberman, I. Y. Misreading: A search for causes. In J. R. Kavanaugh and I. B. Mattingly (Eds.), *Language by ear and by eye*. Cambridge MA: MIT Press, 1972.

Wada, J. Personal communication cited in B. Milner, Hemispheric specialization: Scope and limits. In F.O. Schmitt and F. G. Worden (Eds.), *The neurosciences: Third study program*. Cambridge, MA: MIT Press, 1974.

Wohlwill, J. F. & Wiener, M. Discrimination of form orientation in young children. *Child Development*, 1964, 35, 1113-1125.

Inadequate perception vs. reversals

MARVIN COHN
GEORGE STRICKER

Letter recognition errors may be the result of children going through normal stages of development.

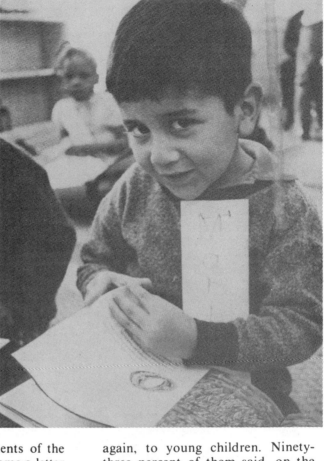

WHEN A child looks at *b* and says *d*, we call this a reversal and infer that the child received a reversed visual image. But how the error occurred is inferred, not observed. It could be the result of many other causes.

A primary reason for concern arises when children are asked to name letters correctly. They must learn to flagrantly violate a previously useful rule which says that spatial orientation is of no value in object identification. Up to now, no matter which way an object (such as a chair or a book) faced, it was still the same object. But suddenly the rule no longer applies when the child looks at letters. Though the letter forms themselves are often identical (*b-d, p-q, u-n*) the names of some letters are completely changed as their spatial orientation varies. As a reflection of the confusion that results when a change in spatial orientation seems to produce a different letter, some children say when looking at *u,* "That's an *n* but it's upside down!" This response suggests that the error has nothing at all to do with receiving a distorted visual image.

A second source of difficulty, apart from perceptual distortion, arises from the components of the letter naming task. To name a letter correctly, the child must first receive the correct visual stimulus, and then must know what name to associate with that stimulus. Why shouldn't a substantial number of letter naming errors come from the latter cognitive area, rather than from the perceptual area? Some children have not as yet learned the names of the letters well, or are not yet sure which name is associated with one of a number of similarly formed letters.

A third source of difficulty is suggested by Piaget, who says that first graders tend to focus attention on a single striking feature of an object, neglecting its other components, which results in inadequate awareness. Even when shown repeatedly that the same amount of water completely fills either a tall thin cylinder or a short, squat one, the children say that one cylinder contains more, either because it is taller or wider than the other one (Flavell, 1963).

As though exploring this in letter recognition, Jackson (1972) showed the letters *b* and *d* in black on clear plastic, at first side by side, then superimposed, and then side by side again, to young children. Ninety-three percent of them said, on the first (side by side) viewing that *b* and *d* were the same. With the letters superimposed (ⱕ), eighty-six percent of the European children and twenty-three percent of the New Guinean children said the letters were different. When the letters were juxtaposed again, seventy-six percent of both groups reverted to their first response, that the two letters were the same. Aren't Jackson's children bearing out Piaget's finding? To the degree that this is so, perceptual reversal is not needed to explain "reversal" errors.

The authors wanted, among other things, to separate the perceptual from the cognitive issues in letter naming. We wanted to know if a child was getting the correct perceptual image when he looked at a letter. For this purpose, an additional test was devised and added to the letter naming task, as follows.

Each child was confronted with a series of twelve "squares," each drawn with one missing side; four examples follow.

⊔ ⊐ ⊓ ⊏

2. DIAGNOSIS AND ASSESSMENT

The twelve "squares" were presented in fixed random order, with each of the sides missing three times. We reasoned that if, for example, a child looked at *b* and reversed its right and left edges so that he saw *d*, he would also reverse the right and left edges of the boxes. Where the right or left side was missing, such a child should indicate that the opposite side was left out. Each child was given a sample row of figures to do first. He was asked to find the open side, and to pretend to draw a line to close it. When the examiner was convinced that the child understood the task, the sample row of "squares" was withdrawn, and the child was asked to close twelve more figures.

Our sample consisted of 409 children, each one of whom "closed" twelve "squares" for a total of 4,908. Result: every single one was done correctly. There were twelve to fifteen apparently anxious children who started correctly and then began to make errors, usually tracing the three closed sides. When stopped, reminded of the directions, and asked to resume the task, even those children then did it all easily, quickly, and correctly.

Why was the square closing task done so much more successfully and easily than the letter naming task? Perhaps because the square closing task relied solely on accurate perception, and did not require any additional cognitive or memory process. Since it was done so universally successfully, this very strongly suggests that the early letter naming difficulties of our sample are not caused by perceptual distortion.

Two studies by Bortner and Birch (1960, 1962), who examined the perceptual performance of clearly brain-injured subjects, support our findings. The Wechsler Intelligence Scale block design subtest was given to hemiplegics and to cerebral palsy patients, who failed eighty-six and eighty-nine items respectively. These experiments proved that 81 percent and 79 percent respectively of even these brain-injured subjects' apparently perceptual errors were not due to perceptual problems, but to motor problems. It seems quite probable that the block design forms are far more complicated than the letter forms we used.

These studies lead to the conclusion that visual discrimination or perception is not a principal source of these individuals' difficulty. Is it likely that nervous system damage or visual perception problems accounted for the letter discrimination errors of the 409 children (several complete classes in normal schools) in our study? We think not!

An examination of the responses and response patterns of our 409 subjects throws further light on the so-called reversal problem. The following list shows the number of correct letter identifications for *b*, *d*, *p*, and *q* in upper and lower case (*N*=409):

Upper case	No. correct	Lower case	No. correct
B	363	b	211
D	311	d	174
P	329	p	320
Q	328	q	38

In upper case, *B*, *D*, *P*, and *Q* are the third, fourteenth, seventh, and eighth easiest letters to identify, respectively. All except *D* are in the easiest third of the alphabet to recognize. Perhaps they are easy to name because spatial orientation is not a problem, since the rounded part of the *B*, *D*, and *P* all go to the right. Further, the rounded parts of these letters do not share the same shape or size, as they do in their lower case counterparts. *Q* in no way resembles the other three.

The same population sample found lower case *b*, *d*, *p*, and *q* the twentieth, twenty-third, sixth, and twenty-sixth easiest letters to name! All but *p* are in the hardest third to identify correctly.

What is it that makes these letters so easy to name correctly in upper case and so hard to identify in lower case? Is auditory perception a factor? The upper case *B*, *D*, *P*, whose names rhyme, are easily named by the children. The lower case *b*, *d*, *p* are easily confused by the same children. Hence we draw two conclusions: 1) Auditory discrimination is not a major factor in the difficulty with naming these letters. 2) The increased difficulty in naming these lower case letters is primarily, if not completely, due to the increased similarity of their visual forms.

Why is the *p* so much easier to name than its three companions? Quite likely because it is the only one of these four letters that has the same general form in upper and lower case (*B*, *b*, *D*, *d*, *P*, *p*, *Q*, *q*). It is less confusing to remember one form for a letter than to remember two. This was clearly demonstrated in a previous study (Cohn, 1976) and in this study.

Why should *q* be so much more difficult to identify than the other three? It is the most difficult letter to recognize, with only thirty-eight of 409 children naming it correctly. It is difficult to argue that children don't know of the existence of the letter, or don't have many opportunities to see it when, in the same population sample, 328 children recognized *Q* in upper case. Evidence is not conclusive on this point.

Are reversal errors commutative (reversible)? If the brain makes a right-to-left reversal of the image of the letter *b*, for example, causing it to appear as *d*, it is reasonable to assume it will make the same reversal when the child looks at *d*, causing it to appear as *b*. Let us examine the evidence on this point.

When our sample looked at *b*, seventy-nine children said *d*. When they looked at *d*, 102 said *b*. However, only twenty children made both these errors. If these children are making right-to-left edge reversals (*b* for *d*, or *d* for *b*), why are they doing it for one letter and not also for the other?

Even more compellingly, one of the present authors previously tested 322 children in lower case alphabet recognition, as well as the 409 in this study. In the total sample of 731 children, 376 looked at *q* and said *p*. *However, none of the children, not a single one, looked at p and said q!* If they suffer from a distortion of perception that transposes the right and left edges of letters, it is a very selective distortion, operating when they look at *q* but not when they look at *p*. Going back to our twenty children who said *d* for *b* as well as *b* for *d*, not one of these looked at *q* and said *p*.

Let us examine further this issue of the commutative quality of reversals. All figures are taken from our second study (*N*=409), the only one for which we have sufficient data to allow us to examine this question.

While twenty-six children looked at *u* and said *n*, thirteen looked at *n* and said *u*. However, only one child (of 409) made both errors.

Sixteen children looked at *m* and said *w*, while twenty-seven looked at *w* and said *m*, but only three children made both errors. One of these three children (the only one in the entire sample), looked at *M* and said *W*, and also looked at *W* and said *M*. *No child was found who consistently rotated or reversed the letters* b, d, p, q, u, n, m, w, M *and* W *in the same direction.*

The evidence above is summarized in four conclusions. 1) No evidence was found to support the concept of consistent direction of reversal within the perception of individual children. 2) The Bortner and Birch studies suggest that even among brain-injured individuals, perceptual distortion is not a major problem. 3) If such consistent perceptual reversal does exist, it will probably be found in only a tiny minority of the population. 4) Although it is common practice to label these errors "reversals," they are product rather than process reversals. In other words, although the letter or product *d*, for example, is the reverse of the letter or product *b*, the process by which the child says one when he looks at the other has nothing to do with perceptual reversal.

We must look instead to other explanations. We had previously mentioned two: 1) the child may not yet have learned the letter names, or may know them, but not yet know which visual letter form to associate them to; 2) the child may not yet have realized that when he looks at certain letters, unlike when he looks at a chair or a person, the name and nature of some letters change as they change position in space.

There is at least a third explanation which we have not as yet discussed. As adults, most of us have mature, normally developed perceptual abilities. However, most of us could not correctly identify the brand name, year, and model name or number of the cars passing on the road outside. Most of us could not identify small variations in different shades of blue with the same ease as a person in charge of mixing dyes at a yarn factory. We have generally ade-

quate perceptual ability, without having developed every conceivable perceptual skill. It is quite possible that children who have normal perceptual ability have not yet used it to develop the skills they need to handle the perceptual part of the letter naming task. They often need more time and experience to learn to do so. And, in point of fact, as children go on through school, their letter recognition difficulties disappear to all practical intents and purposes.

As we look at the letter naming efforts of the samples we studied, we find additional evidence to suggest that undifferentiated perception is responsible for many errors in which reversals could not have played a role. For example, in this study *l* is the second most difficult letter to name, with only seventy-three children getting it right. Most of the errors made in naming this letter were highly systematic, as follows: 170 children said *I* (or *i*); eighty-eight children said "one."

It seems extremely likely that these errors were made because the children observed the obvious long straight line which is the major part of the letter *l*, and based their choice of letter name on it. It also seems extremely likely that some children did not know which of the small, horizontal parts attached to the long vertical line make it a one or an *I* (or an *i*). (In fact many typewriters use the same key for *l* and one.) In the same way, forty-three children looked at *j* and said *I* (or *i*). Again, reversal could not have been an issue. It is probable these children were responding either to the long straight line, or the dot, and based their choice on this single characteristic, rather than on an awareness of all the component parts of the letter and the way in which they are combined. There is also the possibility, of course, that some of the children simply did not know the correct letter name and said the name of the symbol they did know which at least resembled the one they were looking at.

When we examine the errors our sample made in naming any letter, there are always some "I don't know" responses and some letters said only once or a few times each, suggesting that they are random guesses. The other responses are systematic

errors, and are distributed among letters that usually visually resemble the letter to be named.

Our contention is that this kind of unsophisticated perception would also lead to what appears to be reversal errors. All four, *b, d, p, q,* share not one but two and possibly three obvious features—a straight line, a circle, and a relationship of tangency. What differentiates these letter forms from each other is much less obvious, and therefore more confusing (especially to children who have previously learned that objects and people do not change their names, natures, or functions when they face in different directions). The most parsimonious explanation of letter recognition errors is that some children have not yet learned all of the letter names, and others know the names but are not yet sure which name to apply to a given letter form when it visually resembles other letter forms. The idea of consistent perceptual distortion as a major source of difficulty is ruled out on the following grounds:

1) An examination of letter naming errors shows that these errors which should be commutative (reversible) are not.

2) Even in brain-injured populations, visual perception is not the major source of inability to reproduce block designs, as it would be if reversals were present.

3) This study explored whether or not 409 children received visual reversals by asking them to close "squares." These children did not show any reversals or rotations.

4) A more parsimonious explanation has been developed which explains both reversal and non-reversal errors as results of the same processes, and is consistent with careful exploration of the errors actually made. The reversal theory, of course, does not explain non-reversal errors nor is it even consistent with the reversal errors made as explored in this study.

The fact that so many children have trouble in learning to name the letters suggests that we may be trying to teach them before they are maturationally ready to do so. Letter recognition errors appear to be, for the most part, the result of children going through normal stages of development. These stages are gone through more rapidly by some than by others, but by practically all children in the final analysis.

Therefore, these errors should not be seen as a departure from the norm, nor should the children who manifest them be labeled and treated as abnormal individuals saddled with potentially crippling distorted perception. Neither should these children be subjected to special programs designed to correct abnormal perception. There undoubtedly are children with truly distorted perception, but they are probably only a tiny minority of the number thought to be so afflicted.

As a final comment, it seems necessary to reevaluate the perceptual training programs which are used to correct the learning problems of children who manifest "reversals." Training designed to reinforce the concept of constancy of shape is probably counterproductive in that it teaches children that nonsymmetrical forms, such as the triangle, do not acquire new names or characteristics when they are rotated or reversed. That is a principle that will lead to errors when children are trying to identify many of the lower case letters. The apparent success of these programs may well be based on naturally occurring maturational processes, plus the additional learning opportunities that time itself brings.

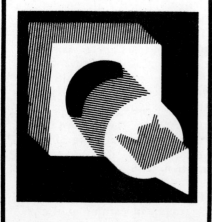

Normal and Disabled Readers Can Locate and Identify Letters: Where's The Perceptual Deficit?

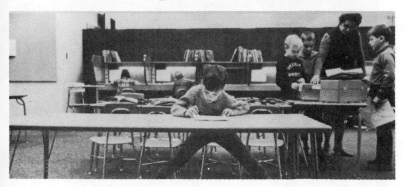

Dennis F. Fisher
Behavioral Research Directorate
U.S. Army Human Engineering Laboratory

Anthony Frankfurter
J.F. Kennedy Institute
Johns Hopkins University

Abstract. In a backward masking letter identification and localization task, performance of children with reading disabilities was compared to that of normal readers matched for age and reading level. On all measures, the performance of the disabled reader group was superior to that of the control groups. This included: correct identification, correct localization, absolute number correct and fewer intrusions. The data are interpreted as indicating that previous hypotheses about visual perceptual difficulties are inadequate in explaining reading disabilities. Alternatively, it is suggested that a reorientation of remedial techniques should be implemented. These should include phonics and graphemic to phonemic encoding, both of which compensate for losses in higher order verbal cognitive processing ability.

Until recently the cause of reading deficiency has been largely attributed to general visual perceptual deficits in form orientation and spatial discriminations (Orton, 1937; Frostig, 1968) and with few exceptions (e.g., Benton, 1962), this position has been left unchallenged. More recently, Kershner (1975), Larsen and Hammill (1975), Stanley, Kaplan and Poole (1975), and Velluntino, Steger and Kandel (1972) found high degrees of comparability between poor and normal reader performance on a variety of perceptual tasks, e.g., spatial transformations and tactile serial matching.

One specific aspect of perceptual processing thought to discriminate disabled and normal readers is maturational lag (Lyle & Goyen, 1975; Satz, Rardin & Ross, 1971) as evidenced in early verbal information processing ability (i.e., within the 250 msec intersaccadic fixation time or iconic storage). Gummerman and Gray (1972) used a backward masking task to limit stimulus processing time and found evidence suggesting that the iconic or brief visual information storage stage in children was longer than that found in older children and adults, but probably only reflected a slower processing speed. Stanley and Hall (1973) found evidence of an extended iconic storage for disabled readers and interpreted the extension as being disruptive to the rate and efficiency with which information was transferred from iconic storage to short-term memory. Although they used a backward masking task to assess group differences at the iconic storage stage, a more appropriate measure would have been a mask versus no-mask comparison as Gummerman and Gray have used. To complicate matters further, Katz and Wicklund (1972) found age differences, but no differences between good and poor readers within grades, on a letter scanning task. Taken together, these data might be interpreted as indicating that maturational factors which distinguish iconic storage at different grade levels may differ substantially from those that characterize iconic storage in good and poor readers.

The present experiment will examine three possible deficits in early visual information processing which may account for reading disability. These are: a general perceptual deficit, which should be witnessed by overall poorer performance on the part of the disabled reader group, and particularly on letter identification and localization; a maturational lag, which should be evidenced by the similar performance of older disabled readers and younger reading level matched children; and the extended iconic storage, which should be reflected in larger masking versus no-masking performance differences for the disabled reader as compared to the control groups. The number of letters corrently identified and located by children matched in reading and age level to disabled readers, under both backward masking and no-masking conditions, will be compared.

METHOD

Subjects. Three groups of 12 children served as subjects. Group 1 was comprised of 12 children from the Kennedy School, J.F. Kennedy Institute of the Johns Hopkins University. These children were diagnosed as disabled readers (dyslexics)[b] and were undergoing intensive remediation. Their mean age was 10 years 8 months (s.d. = .84) and reading level was equivalent to grade 2.8 (s.d. = .55) on the Gates-Mac-Ginitie Vocabulary Test. These children were performing at or above their appropriate grade level on non-verbal, e.g., arithmetic skills. Groups 2 and 3 were children matched to Group 1 by reading level and age, respectively. Reading level matched children were from grades 2 and 3 with reading grade equivalent of 2.5 (s.d. = .86) on Gates-MacGinitie Vocabulary Test, at the Bakersfield Elementary School, Aberdeen, Maryland. Age level matched children were from grades 5 and 6 (mean age = 10 years 8 months; s.d. = .92) at Aberdeen Middle School, Aberdeen, Maryland. Both reading level and age level matched children were judged to be at or above average reading level and mental ability by their teachers. In all cases parental permission was received prior to each child's participation.

Stimuli and Sequencing. Stimuli were the upper case angular letters: F, H, N, V, W, X and Z. On each trial, 2, 4, or 6 of these letters were presented randomly in a 16 cell (4x4) matrix. Each stimulus array was exposed to the subjects for 200 msec. Each letter and cell were used equally often for each stimulus array size. The matrices were presented by rear projection, 140 cm from the subject, subtending a visual angle of 2.45° square, while each letter subtended .3° vertically. The stimuli were presented in rooms that were dimly lit at a luminance of approximately 70 Cd/m^2. A dark fixation point marked the center of the matrix. Stimuli and masks were presented by Kodak Carousel Projectors while the synchrony and duration were controlled by Massey-Dickinson Co. Timers and Electronic Shutters. In one of the two sessions a mask composed of a dense and jumbled group of letter fragments (following the guidelines of Haber, 1970) occurred immediately following the 200 msec stimulus

[b]For our purposes the terms *dyslexic* and *disabled reader* are taken to mean those who have failed, by at least 2 years, to achieve normal grade level reading skills for reasons other than emotional instability, intellectual deficiency, or brain injury.

exposure. The mask was presented within the normal time frame of the iconic storage stage, in accord with the assumption that the contours of the mask in some way interfere with the contours of the letters in the stimulus arrray, thereby limiting processing time.

Procedure. Each child participated individually in two sessions, each lasting approximately 30 min. and separated by 24 hours. During each session the children were instructed to look at a dot on the screen which marked the center of the stimulus array. When the children indicated "ready" the array was flashed to them. The children were given sets of blank matrices on which they were instructed to write down the letters they saw and the location in which each occurred. Each child was given practice and familiarity with the stimulus set and mask - no-mask procedures. Each session consisted of 72 trials, 24 at each of 2, 4, and 6 item array sizes presented in random order. Additional practice was given to any child who needed it. Half of the participants received the mask trials first, and other half received the no-mask trials first.

RESULTS

The data were subjected to 2 x 2 x 3 analyses of variance, with groups as a between-effect and mask - no-mask and stimulus array sizes (2, 4, or 6 letters) as within-effects. Of particular interest in defining group differences will be a discussion of the following measures: correct letter; correct location; correct letter — correct location; and intrusions. For each of these measures only those effects which discriminate the groups will be discussed. That is, the main effects of mask - no-mask and stimulus array size were highly significant beyond the .01 level in all analyses, but are of little theoretical interest because they do not discriminate between the groups. Therefore, mask and array size effects will be discussed only if they interact with the groups effect. No analysis performed reflected effects of presentation order, i.e., no-mask condition first of second, and therefore further reference will be omitted. In general, these data will be described in terms of number correct out of 48, 96 and 144 possible per session for the 2, 4, and 6 element arrays, respectively.

Correct Letters

The analysis of correct letters reported (irrespective of location) revealed a significant main effect for groups, $F(2, 33) = 19.1$, $p < .01$ and a significant interaction of Array Size x Groups, $F(4, 66) = 6.3$, $p < .001$. The data for the main effect and interaction are shown in Table 1. In short, although all groups improved as the array size increased, the rate of increase and overall number of correct letters reported were greater for the disabled readers. In addition, a significant interaction of Mask x Groups, $F(2, 33) = 5.3$, $p < .01$ was found and these data are shown in Figure 1. From this figure it can be seen that the absence of a mask led to a much greater increase in performance for the reading and age level groups than for the disabled readers. No other interaction involving groups reached the .05 level of significance.

Table 1
Mean Number of Correct Letters Identified* per Session

	ARRAY SIZE				
	2	4	6	$\tilde{X}$	[% Diff. 2-6]
Disabled	34.2 (71)	498. (52)	64.2 (45)	49.5	(26)
Age	30.3 (63)	42.3 (44)	51.3 (35)	41.4	(28)
Reading	23.1 (48)	27.6 (29)	33.0 (23)	27.9	(25)

*percent of total in parentheses

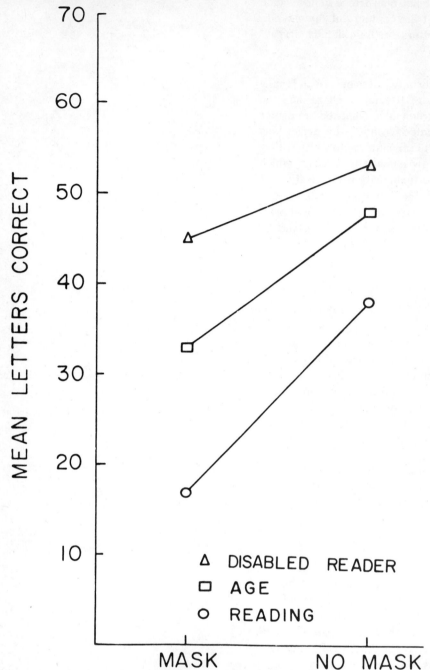

Figure 1. Mean letters correct as a function of mask and no-mask conditions for the three groups.

A subsequent analysis comparing the disabled and age level matched groups again revealed a significant difference between these two groups, $F(1, 22) = 4.48$, $p < .05$. In addition, the interaction of Mask x Groups, $F(2, 44) = 6.20$, $P< .01$, also proved significant, possibly indicating a longer iconic storage stage in normal readers. No other interactions involving groups for the secondary analysis reached the .05 level of significance.

These data are interpreted as failing to support general perceptual deficit or maturational lag notions in that letter identification was found to be better for the disabled readers than the two control groups. The hypothesis of inefficient processing out of the icon due to its extended duration also fails to receive support. In fact, the curves in figure 1 show the difference between mask and no-mask conditions to be smallest for the disabled readers, quite contrary to expectancy. It should also be noted from Table 1 that the percentages of total possible correct responses decrease with increasing trial length. Most notable, the percentage difference or drop in accuracy performance between the two and six array sizes is consistent for all three groups. No difference was found between age level match and disabled readers as a function or array size.

Correct Location

The analysis of correct location (irrespective of letter entered) yielded a significant main effect for groups, $F(2, 33) = 21.3$, p $< .001$ with means of 44.4, 26.1 and 36.0 locations reported correctly per session and across array size for the disabled, reading and age level groups, respectively. A significant interaction of Mask x Groups, $F(2, 33) = 4.4$, p $< .05$ was found, indicating once again that the no-mask condition was more beneficial to the reading and age level groups than the disabled readers. In addition, the interactions of Mask x Array Size, $F(2. 66) = 6.5$, p $< .01$ and Mask x Array Size x Groups, $F(4,66) = 2.64$, p $< .05$ indicate that performance not only increased in the no-mask

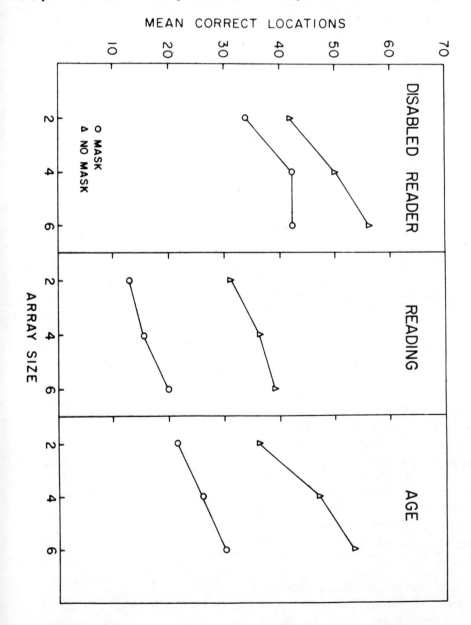

Figure 2. Mean locations correct as a function of mask and no-mask conditions and array size for the three groups.

condition differentially for the three groups, but reporting location information improved differentially as a function of array size between mask and no-mask conditions. The data for this latter interaction are shown in Figure 2. No other main effects or interactions involving groups reached the .05 level of significance.

A subsequent analysis comparing only the disabled and age level matched group again showed a significant main effect for groups, $F(1,22) = 6.58$, p < .05 and a significant Groups x Mask interaction, $F(2,44) = 10.1$, p < .01. As in the analysis for correct letters this analysis failed to reveal an Array Size x Groups effect, indicating that the primary contribution to the array size effect comes from the reading level matched groups, which are then both quantitatively and qualitatively different from either of the other older age groups.

Again, these data fail to support any of the three alternative explanations for reading disability. More importantly, however, is the fact that these data indicate that the disabled readers can spatially organize visual verbal information.

Correct Letter — Correct Location

The analysis of correct letter — correct location represents the most stringent criterion for these data analyses. In order for a correct response to be scored, a letter must have been identified and located as it appeared in the stimulus array. This analysis yielded a significant main effect for groups, $F(2,33) = 10.5$, p < .01 and a significant interaction of Array Size x Groups, $F(4,66) = 5.16$, p < .01. The data for this interaction and main effect are shown in Table 2. From this table it can be seen that the performance of the disabled readers decreased with increasing array size, this was not the case for the other two groups. No other discriminating main effects or interactions were obtained in this analysis.

Table 2
Mean Number of Correct Letters Identified - Located* per session

	ARRAY SIZE				
	2	4	6	$\bar{X}$	[% Diff. 2-6]
Disabled	27.8 (58)	26.8 (28)	24.3 (17)	26.2	(41)
Age	22.2 (47)	24.0 (25)	24.5 (17)	23.8	(30)
Reading	16.3 (34)	17.8 (18)	17.3 (12)	16.7	(22)

*percent of total in parentheses

A secondary analysis was performed on these data, once again comparing the disbaled readers to age level matches. No main effect difference was found between these groups (F = 1.0, n.s.), however, the interaction of Array Size x Groups, $F(2,44) = 7.4$, p < 01, was maintained from the overall analysis. This interaction indicates that as the array sizes became more complex, the disabled readers became increasingly less able to correctly identify and locate items in the array. More importantly, however, is the fact that even though they do show a decrease in performance they still operate at the level of their age level matches. It is also interesting to note that for all groups across array sizes performance remained relatively stable, but does reflect substantial decreases in percentage of correct responses due to the higher number correct possible in the six item arrays.

In short, these data do not support a general perceptual deficit hypothesis, by virtue of the equivalent performance shown by the disabled group, or a maturational lag hypothesis as the disabled readers out-performed the reading level matched group. In addition, when the most extreme criterion of correct performance was applied to these data, no masking vs. no-masking effects were found. It is as though all the identification — location information is most accurately retrieved during the time prior to the mask and all other information taken in after that time suffers *both* in identity or location accuracy.

Intrusions [Incorrect Letter — Incorrect Location]

Intrusions were letter responses that were not included in the stimulus set and were placed in cells of the response matrix not occupied by items in the stimulus array. The analysis of variance failed to reveal a groups effect, F < 1.0, however, the groups did differ as a function of array size as indicated by the significant interaction of Array Size x Groups, $F(4,66) = 6.76, P < .01$. These data are shown in Table 3, and represent a range of .12 to .4 letters per trial. The reasons for the irregularities, e.g., high number of intrusions in the four item array for the disabled group, are yet unexplainable, however, little relevance is seen as applicable to any of the three alternative explanations for reading disability.

Table 3
Mean Number of Intrusions

Groups	ARRAY SIZE		
	2	4	6
Disabled	3.6	9.6	3.2
Reading	9.2	7.6	5.3
Age	6.1	7.5	2.8

DISCUSSION

The results from this experiment can be summarized as follows: the reading disabled group made more correct responses than groups matched for age and reading level. In short, these data provide no evidence for a general perceptual decrement either at the graphemic identification or spatial localization level. Moreover, group comparisons failed to support a maturational lag hypothesis or a specific perceptual decrement at the iconic storage level as the disabled readers always outperformed their reading level matched counterparts.

The most stringent analysis (correct letter — correct location), revealed that the disabled readers and age level matches performed equivalently overall, but the disabled group performance decreased slightly, though significantly, over array sizes while the control groups increased slightly. We might speculate that such a decrease is evidence of a limitation of memorial processes rather than of perceptual processes. That is, analyses for correct letter and correct location revealed increasing performance trends (percentage decreases were equivalent) as array size increased. This performance was not dependent upon absolute identity with the stimulus array, but simply one of identifying letters and locations which the disabled group was able to do quite well. For absolute accuracy, the disabled readers' iconic storage is as durable as the age level matches, but output seems less restrained by absolute accuracy considerations.

The data for correct letter identification as a function of mask condition were shown in Figure 2. Although the disabled readers generally provides more correct letter responses, the differences in the curves seem to indicate that the disabled readers shows less of a mask to no-mask performance difference which goes *contrary* to expectancy for hypotheses attributing performance decrements of reading disability to the iconic storage stage. That is, the longer the iconic storage the greater the expected differences between the no-mask and mask conditions. Longer icons should result in less efficient transfer of information from iconic to short-term memory (Stanley & Hall, 1973). Similar trends are found in the correct location data shown in Figure 2. Taken together these data provide little support for notions aimed at locating the cause of the memory deficit in the previous analysis at the iconic storage stage, but permit such deficits to be at higher order processing stages.

Historically, the disabled reader was consistently shown to be inferior to normal reader control groups regardless of the task involved. The present experiment represents one exception. Another is Katz and Wicklund (1972). They have recently shown that on search and matching tasks little or no performance decrements are found between disabled and normal readers making physical feature matches. The primary locus of difficulty seemed to be at higher order processing stages where naming, i.e., articulating or phonological encoding, was necessitated.

A high incidence of poor naming ability has also been found in poor readers by: Mackworth and Mackworth (1974); Mattis, French and Rapin (1973); and Spring and Capps (1974). Kolers (1975) found poor graphemic pattern-analyzing performance on the part of poor readers, but he interpreted these data as indicative of difficulty more cognitive, i.e., "interpreting and graphemes as linguistic marks", than perceptual.

There is the possibility that having been through a great deal of remediation, including simple graphemic identification, the disabled readers experienced a task-training advantage. Such a possibility exists, but adds *nothing* to a perceptual deficit hypothesis - perceptual processes are intact. Each of the disabled readers in the present experiment could easily identify individual letters, but when letters are to be put together and need to be named as in reading, processing becomes more difficult and less efficient. That is, b is identifed as b, and a is identified as a. But, when b and a are put together in close proximity the disabled reader has a great deal of difficulty identifying ba, and even more difficulty with the longer word *bakery*.

In effect, the performance of the disabled readers may reflect another type of developmental lag. That is, they may tend to treat visual verbal material as singular items and not as units. Multiple element arrays such as those experienced in the present experiment are processed as multiple single items which are not integrated into units. Words such as multiple item arrays are dealt with letter-by-letter and are not unitized. The task employed in the present experiment lended itself very nicely to a letter-by-letter processing strategy. Integration of the information was not required. It is highly likely that both the age and reading level matched groups have already advanced to a more integrative reading strategy and are therefore less able to deal appropriately with individual stimulus materials as presented. If two or more letters were in each of the array cells, or the letters in the two, four and six letter arrays spelled two, four and six letter words, we might well expect the disabled reader group to show vastly inferior performance based on naming ability, than the normal reader control groups.

Meaningful sequences may not be the only requirement. Spring and Farmer (1975) found reduced perceptual spans and naming speed in poor readers compared to normal readers following 250 msec exposures. On the basis of the horizontally displayed digit sequence, which may well force subjects into a left to right scanning strategy involving both temporal and spatial output considerations, we are in agreement with their model "attributing narrow perceptual span to slow phonological coding." McLeod (1967) found that disabled readers were consistently inferior to normal controls in reproducing random letter sequences, but no interaction was found across 0, 1st or 2nd orders of approximation to English. The comparability of his task to the present experiment is not direct as displays were horizontally displayed and were exposed for 1 sec. While no data were reported as a function of varying array sizes or performance on real word sequences the exposure duration seems to allow for the possibility that verbal memorial limitations were discriminating between the groups rather than more perceptual limitations tested by the present experiment.

Obviously, the present task was *not* reading, but it did allow for an assessment of the basic perceptual processes of identification and localization without linguistic or phonological constraints. Differences found in the present experiment were in favor, for the most part, of the disabled readers. These data discredit perceptual difficulties as the cause of reading deficiency. It is hypothesized that the most probable cause of reading disability is a developmental lag which is cognitively based, at the level of naming or translating graphological to phonological information, rather than perceptually based. We find this interpretation in consonance with the findings of Kershner (1975). Larsen and Hammill (1975) have recently taken an even stronger stand in a fine critical review by failing to find any relationship between visual perceptual ability and learning.

We, therefore, advocate a reorientation and reevaluation of present instructional practices. This reorientation should be away from perceptual and perceptual-motor training techniques and toward a greater direct emphasis on word related skills with emphasis on phonics training, orthographic regularity and irregularity, and graphemic to phonemic correspondence. It is unlikely that the severely disabled reader will ever become a reader per se, but through such training word repetoire and recognition skill should be greatly enhanced.

REFERENCES

BENTON, A. Dyslexis in relation to form perception and directional sense. In *Reading Disability: Progress and Research Needs in Dyslexia.* J. Money (Ed.), Baltimore: Johns Hopkins Press, 1962.

FROSTIG, M. Visual modality, research and practice. In H. K. Smith (Ed.), *Perception and Reading*, International Reading Association, 1968, Newark, Delaware, P. 25-33.

GUMMERMAN, K. & GRAY, C. R. Age, iconic storage, and visual information processing. *Journal of Experimental Child Psychology,* 1972, *13,* 165-170,

HABER, R.N. A note on how to choose a mask. *Psychological Bulletin,* 1970, *74,* 373-376.

KATZ, L. & WICKLUND, D. A. Letter scanning rate for good and poor readers in grades two and six. *Journal of Educational Psychology,* 1972, *63,* 363-367.

KERSHNER, J. R. Visual-spatial organization and reading: Support for a cognitive-developmental interpretation. *Journal of Learning Disabilities,* 1975, *8,* 9-16.

KOLERS, P. A. Pattern-analyzing disability in poor readers. *Developmental Psychology,* 1975, *11,* 282-290.

LARSEN, S. C. & HAMMILL, D. C. The relationship of selected visual perceptual abilities to school learning. *Journal of Special Education,* 1975, *9,* 281-291.

LYLE, J. G. & GOYEN, J. D. Effect of speed of exposure and difficulty of discrimination of visual recognition of retarded readers. *Journal of Abnormal Psychology,* 1975, *84,* 673-676.

MACHWORTH, J. F. & MACKWORTH, N. H. How children read: Matching by sight and sound. *Journal of Reading Behavior,* 1974, *6,* 295-303.

MATTIS, S., FRENCH, J.H., & RAPIN, I. Dyslexia in children and young adults — 3 independent neurophysiological syndromes. *Developmental Medicine,* 1973, *17,* 150-163.

McLEOD, J. Some psycholinguistic correlates of reading disability in young children. *Reading Research Quarterly,* 1967, ·2, 5-31.

ORTON, S. T. *Reading, Writing and Speech Problems in Children.* New York: W. W. Norton and Company, 1937.

SATZ, P., RARDIN, D. & ROSS, J. An evaluation of a theory of specific development dyslexia. *Child Development,* 1971, *42,* 2009-2021.

SPRING, C. & CAPPS, C. Encoding speed, rehearsal, and probed recall of dyslexic boys. *Journal of Educational Psychology,* 1974, *66,* 780-786.

SPRING, C. & FARMER, R. Perceptual span of poor reader. *Journal of Reading Behavior,* 1975, *7,* 297-305.

STANLEY, G. & HALL, R. A comparison of dyslexics and normals in recalling letter arrays after brief presentation. *British Journal of Psychology,* 1973, *43,* 301-304.

STANLEY, G., KAPLAN, I., & POOLE, C. Cognitive and non-verbal perceptual processing in dyslexics. *Journal of General Psychology,* 1975, *93,* 67-72.

VELLUNTINO, F. R., STEGER, J. A., & KANDEL, G. Reading disability: An investigation of the perceptual deficit hypothesis. *Cortex,* 1972, *8,* 106-118.

I lev w...
dig hus wi...
my moerth...
and faher.
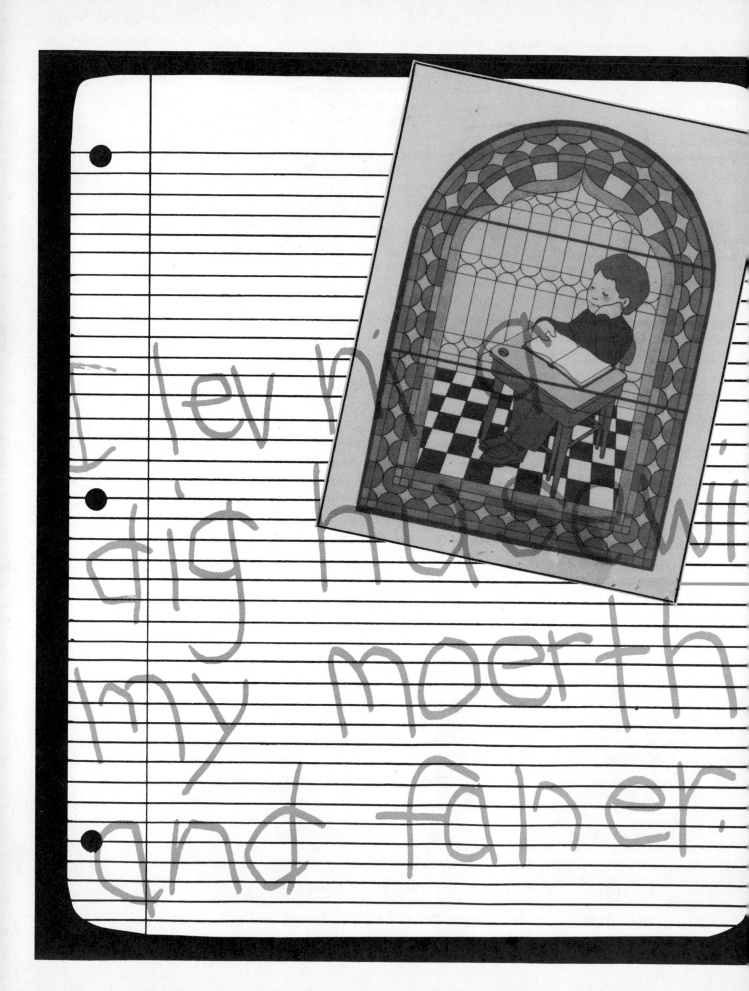

Instructional Techniques

Conventional methods of classroom teaching and training offer little help to dyslexic students. Alternative approaches must be specially designed for them. The first step involves standard and informal testing to help indicate a general diagnosis, pointing out specific strengths and weaknesses of relative perceptual modalities.

The student's academic level is considered in selection of working materials, along with factors of his visual, auditory and tactile modalities so that his program of learning is truly individual to his own needs.

Analysis of observed reading skills most often provide the following important evaluative information:
1. Does the child utilize word analysis skills?
2. What is the extent of his vocabulary?
3. What pattern of consistent word analysis errors occur?
4. Are certain words or parts of words constantly omitted or distorted?

The linguistic approach can then be designed to remediate any of these observed deficiencies. Other approaches include a language experience approach, where the student dictates a story to the teacher, thus making a self experienced story his first step in the process of reading skills. Multi-sensory approaches also offer alternatives to stimulation of learning.

Much is yet to be learned regarding dyslexia and reading disabilities. Special teacher training and new research bring us much needed help in an area which has perplexed educators and the medical profession, but which continues to strive for new methods of treatment through extensive analysis and innovation.

Behavior Therapy of an Eleven-Year-Old Girl with Reading Problems

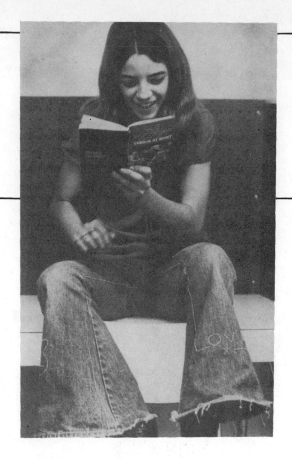

Penny Word and Vitali Rozynko, Ph.D.

A recent behavioral technique, developed to eliminate unwanted behavior, is desensitization (Wolpe 1958). This procedure initially was utilized to countercondition fears (phobias) of specific objects or situations — such as fear of snakes, spiders, heights, closed spaces, etc. Later extensions of this method included its use to alleviate discomfort in talking and socializing with others (Kraft 1969). In this procedure the subject learns to relax, or to behave in a way that is incompatible with autonomic responses associated with the fear response. By engaging in behaviors incompatible with anxiety, the association or connection between the stimulus and the resulting fear response is broken.

A number of researchers and therapists (Ellis 1963, Staats 1972) have concentrated on changing *verbal* behavior — that is, what a person thinks and says. Staats has emphasized that changing verbal behavior has to be considered in conjunction with any plan to change behavior. Language apparently performs a whole series of functions for the individual. Among other things, the verbal system that a person possesses determines what he sees or hears, how he evaluates what he sees or hears, and how he evaluates himself and others. It also controls, or at least influences, what a person

will do in any particular situation. For example, if a person talks to himself or evaluates himself negatively, he is likely to become depressed or anxious. Similarly, if he blames others, he is likely to express anger when he comes into contact with them. Altering the way a person talks to himself (thinks) about himself and others, will assist him in coping with difficult interpersonal situations.

In this case report, the therapy or relearning experience was implemented, with the central focus on the use of relaxation and desensitization. A provocative aspect of this case report is that the techniques of relaxation and desensitization were successful in the modification of a fear response which was directly responsible for a severe reading difficulty in a child.

PROCEDURE

Therapy was begun with an eleven-year-old girl (Eileen) because of severe reading problems she had been manifesting in school. Eileen's parents were concerned with her poor reading and with her continuing nervousness and irritability after school. They consented to behavioral treatment when it was offered.

The therapy was performed in the therapist's home. Since Eileen was a neighbor who had already visited the therapist on several occasions, the time required to build rapport was

"Behavior Therapy of an Eleven-year-old Girl With Reading Problems," Penny Word, Vitali Rozynko, Ph.D., *Journal of Learning Disabilities*, Vol. 7 No. 9, November 1974. ©1974 The Professional Press, Inc.

minimal. Ten sessions, ranging from one-half to one and one-half hours, were given twice each week for five weeks. During the first session, the therapist talked to Eileen specifically about her reading and school problems. Eileen found it difficult to discuss her school problems, but confirmed her parent's report that she was afraid of participating in reading group. In a previous class, the teacher had raised her hand as if she were going to strike Eileen and had made a wry face whenever Eileen stumbled in her reading. Eileen somewhat reluctantly agreed that it might be a good idea if she could learn how to read out loud in her reading group. Eileen was then told what she and the therapist would do over the next several meetings — namely, learn to relax, help to write a story about reading in school, listen to the story that was written, and do some reading. (The word "story" was used rather than "desensitization hierarchy" because it was more understandable to the child.) Toward the end of the first session, Eileen was asked to lie down on a bed and listen to the therapist who proceeded to read aloud a 30-minute relaxation script. After the relaxation period, Eileen was visibly less active and less verbal.

The second session consisted of spending a short time talking with Eileen about her school and in reading the relaxation script. The child's response to the script was similar to her response in the first session.

In the third session, the therapist composed the following "story" (desensitization hierarchy), with Eileen's cooperation:

HAPPINESS IS READING A BOOK
A Story for Eileen

You don't like reading in school. When you were in Mrs. ____'s class, you were punished for not doing what the teacher liked. Now you feel uncomfortable when you must read in school. You are right, but so is the teacher. You could not behave in any other way than you do in reading group. Reading can be fun. You can learn to be comfortable and enjoy learning to read.

(1) Vividly imagine it is Christmas time and you get a package in the mail. You open it and discover a brand new book. You are calm and relaxed.

(2) Vividly imagine you are in class and see Linda, Steve, Christie, Belinda, and Scott sitting in the class room library reading. You are calm and relaxed.

(3) Vividly imagine it is 15 minutes before reading. You are sitting at your desk, doing your sheets. You think about reading. You are calm and relaxed.

(4) Vividly imagine it is reading time; you pick up your book and paper, and go sit down in the reading circle. You are calm and relaxed.

(5) Vividly imagine you are sitting in the reading circle now, and the teacher says, "OK, Eileen." You are calm and relaxed.

(6) Vividly imagine you are sitting in class reading out loud. You are calm and relaxed.

(7) Vividly imagine you come across a word you don't know. You are calm and relaxed.

(8) Vividly imagine you have a substitute teacher, and it is reading time. You lose your place. The teacher gives you a mean look. You are calm and relaxed.

(9) Vividly imagine you have a substitute teacher, and she asks you to read. You make a mistake. The teacher says, "What's wrong with you? Can't you read anything right?" You are calm and relaxed.

(10) Vividly imagine you have a substitute teacher, and it is reading time. You are reading and come to a word you don't know. The teacher looks at you angrily and raises her arm as if she were going to strike you. You are calm and relaxed.

After this story was written, the therapist again read the relaxation script — shortened at Eileen's request to about 15 minutes. After the relaxation period, Eileen asked for help in making a library poster upon which she wrote, "Happiness Is Reading."

The presentation of the "story" (hierarchy items) began in the fourth session. The therapist read the relaxation script and then presented the first six items of the hierarchy. After presentation of the items, Eileen was instructed to imagine a pleasant scene which she and the therapist previously had selected. Upon completion of this session, Eileen picked up a child's book from the table and began to read to the therapist.

The therapist gradually presented all of the ten items in the hierarchy. In the evening at home, after the session in which item #9 was presented ("The teacher says, 'What's wrong with you? Can't you read anything right?'"), Eileen became very upset and told her mother that hearing these words really bothered her. The hierarchy (including the ninth item) was repeated in subsequent sessions until Eileen reported that none of the hierarchy items were disturbing to her.

RESULTS

Eileen's behavior changed in several respects

during the treatment period. Prior to the therapy, Eileen had been restless, demanding, and extremely talkative. After the first two relaxation sessions, her rate of talking dropped drastically. She became much less distractible, and was able to persist on tasks for much longer periods of time without having to ask for help. Eileen apparently liked relaxing, and her mother reported, toward the seventh or eighth session, that Eileen would ask her to read the relaxation script to her after a particularly difficult day in school.

Prior to the relaxation-desensitization sequence, when Eileen was visiting the therapist on an informal basis, she had become angry when the therapist picked up a book to read. She also had refused to read and had criticized any book offered to her, saying it was "boring" or "no good." In school, Eileen had refused to read out loud in the reading group and had been receiving failing grades in reading. After the fourth relaxation-desensitization session, Eileen, without prompting, picked up a book and started to read aloud. The therapist made no attempt to correct any mistakes that she made, and told Eileen how much she enjoyed having her read to her. From the fourth session on, Eileen came to visit the therapist between sessions just to read to her. Eileen continued these intersession visits until after the relaxation-desensitization procedures had been completed. Around the time of the seventh session, Eileen told the therapist she was going to the library. Her mother's reports indicated that Eileen began going to the library at least twice each week and brought home at least two books each time.

In the ninth session, Eileen told the therapist that she no longer was afraid of the reading group, and the relaxation-desensitization procedure was terminated following the tenth session. The therapist did not keep any records of reading improvement during this time, but at the end of the semester, Eileen received a satisfactory grade in reading — an improvement over her previous grade which had been "needs to improve." The teacher also noted that Eileen had shown an increased interest in all of her work. A year after the treatment was completed, the therapist received a "thank you" letter from Eileen, which also said that she was now in the fifth grade and reading on the fifth grade level. Prior to therapy, Eileen had been reading at a level below most of her classmates.

DISCUSSION

Eileen's reading problem seemed to have been associated with a series of punishing experiences at school. Because of these experiences Eileen avoided reading, and felt extremely uncomfortable in situations where others were reading. Her disparaging remarks about books and reading, in general, may have served to alleviate her discomfort in reading situations.

The therapist utilized relaxation and desensitization techniques to reduce the fear response and concomitantly reinforced the behaviors of reading and talking positively about reading.

The immediate effect of the first two sessions of relaxation training was striking, and it is likely that it made possible the "cooperative" writing of the "story" of hierarchy items (third session) by reducing the child's general level of anxiety and the rate of her avoidance responses. Constructing the hierarchy had a multiple function. In order for the story to be, Eileen had to talk about experiences which obviously were uncomfortable for her. The story was written using many of her own words which she had to repeat several times, and consequently she was imagining the frightening situations. Thus, by the time formal desensitization procedures had begun, some unlearning and adaptation had already occurred. In addition, the story also provided an alternative method of talking about reading which the child may have repeated again after the session in titling her poster, "Happiness Is Reading."

The desensitization procedure presented little difficulty to the child, and she completed the 10-item hierarchy in a total of eight sessions. Simultaneously, the therapist provided Eileen with the opportunity to practice her reading. In this situation, the therapist praised her for her reading and did not correct or criticize her for her mistakes. In effect, counterconditioning was proceeding: the behavior of reading was followed by positive reinforcement and not punishment or criticism.

Eileen's reading difficulties were a function of learned dysfunctional avoidance responses as opposed to difficulties in encoding. It is likely that many children experience reading or other learning difficulties because of having received criticism from teachers, parents, or peers. In some cases, these children may read only with difficulty and, in others, such experiences may even prevent the learning of initial reading behaviors. For such children, some consideration might be given to instituting procedures to unlearn fear or avoidance responses associated with reading prior to beginning formal remedial training. Relaxation training may prove extremely helpful and, in some cases, desensitization techniques may be appropriate.

This case report is anecdotal and presents clinical observations and reports from the child, her parents, and teacher as evidence of effectiveness. The specific techniques used in the treatment have not been reported in the literature on treatment of reading difficulties. This case report might be considered exploratory but seminal.

No additional objective data are available regarding reading rates, anxiety levels, and even client characteristics. Any teacher trying this technique should obtain objective pre- and post-therapy measures in these areas to determine the effectiveness of the method with any client or group of clients. This paper, however, serves to point the way toward a possibly fruitful area for future research in the modification of reading and other school-related learning problems. Future research must be in the areas of effectiveness of the relaxation-desensitization approach on different populations, persons with different types of learning problems, and on children with different background characteristics. Future studies also need to specify clearly the technique used and to differentiate more clearly the effects of relaxation, and reinforcement. *Veterans Administration Hospital, 3801 Miranda Avenue, Palo Alto, Calif. 94304.*

REFERENCES
Ellis, A.: *Reason and Emotion in Psychotherapy.* New York: Lyle-Stuart, 1963.
Kraft, T.: *Alcoholism treated by systematic desensitization: A follow-up of eight cases. J. Roy, Coll. Gen. Pract., 1969, 18, 336-340.*
Staats, A.W.: *Language behavior therapy: A derivative of social behaviorism. Behav. Ther., 1972, 3, 165-192.*
Wolpe, J.: *Psychotherapy by Reciprocal Inhibition.* Stanford Univ. Press, 1958.

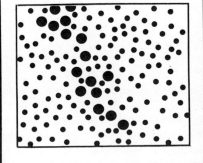

A "Sweep" Procedure For Reading Improvement

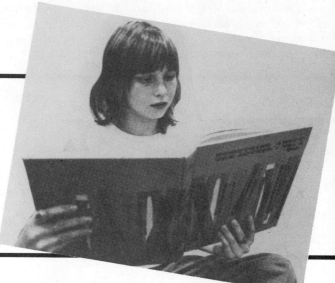

DAVID RYBACK
West Georgia College, Carrollton, Georgia 30117

A simply-administered yet highly effective procedure for reading improvement was tested on a ten-year-old dyslexic child. The procedure involves covering a word with the right thumb and slowly revealing the word while encouraging the child in phonetic mastery. Three separate reading tests indicated that the procedure was highly effective in teaching phonetic aspects of reading as opposed to other general reading skills including speed in reading.

There is always a strong interest in more effective approaches to teaching reading skills. The procedure described here was developed by the present author over eight years ago while teaching reading skills to autistic children, but this study represents the first attempt at systematic observation of the procedure as used with a dyslexic child.

The subject in this study was a ten-year-old boy in the fourth grade of school, reading at the second grade level. He obtained a verbal score of 87 and a performance score of 97 on the Wechsler Intelligence Scale for Children, for a full scale score of 91.

The Ryback Sweep Procedure can be characterized as a phonetic approach in which the child is taught to read phonetically at his own pace by covering the difficult word with his right thumb and by sounding out the letters as he gradually uncovers the word by moving his thumb to the right. The child is of course first taught to sound out letters in a conventional manner, if this is necessary. During the initial phase of training, the teacher uses her own right thumb to slowly uncover the target word, as she correspondingly sounds out the part of the word being revealed from under her thumb. During this phase, the child learns to read phonetically while the teacher sweeps the word. Gradually, however, the child is taught to "sweep" on his own while the teacher corrects and encourages when necessary.

The advantages of this surprising simple procedure is that it entails no special equipment or material, yet makes use of the scanning procedure available, typically, with costly mechanical apparatus. Hence, it is easily available to all teachters and their students.

As well, it gives the dyslexic child an opportunity to gain a sense of self-mastery as he learns to sweep words on his own, at his own pace. In addition, once the habit is strongly ingrained during the final phase, the child eventually learns to sweep, i.e. scan, words phonetically without use of his thumb and so becomes independent of even the last overt vestige of any technique and can now see himself as reading normally without aid. This enhances significantly his sense of mastery over his reading problem and improves his motivation for further development in reading skills.

In order to examine the child's progress fully, three tests of reading were employed during the two months of training—the Slosson Oral Reading Test, the Wide Range Achievement Test, and the Gray Oral Reading Test. Each of the tests was administered before training was initiated, after one month of training, and at the end of two months of training. Results of testing were indicated in Table 1.

Different results were obtained with each of the tests. The Slosson is a good indication of phonetic reading skills and showed over one year's progress after the first month of training and an additional

"A 'Sweep' Procedure for Reading Improvement," David Ryback, *Reading Improvement*, Vol. 13 No. 2, Summer 1976. ©1976 Project Innovation.

TABLE 1
Reading Progress According to the Slosson Oral Reading Test,
Wide Range Achievement Test, and Gray Oral Reading Test

Time of Administration	Reading Grade Level		
	SORT	WRAT	GORT
Prior to training	1.6	2.1	1.9
After one month of training	2.6	2.3	1.9
After two months of training	3.8	2.6	1.9

year's progress after the second month of training. The WRAT, a general test of reading skills, showed 2 months of reading progress after the first month of training and an additional 3 months of progress after the second month of training. The Gray Oral, sensitive to reading speed, indicated no progress at all during the two months of training.

The over-all results of the three tests indicated that the Ryback Sweep Procedure proved extremely effective in aiding the child's acquisition of phonetic reading skills, as opposed to non-phonetic reading skills. However, the child's reading speed was not improved.

As previously indicated, the Ryback Sweep Procedure does not involve any apparatus or particular reading material and can be easily taught to teachers and parents.

Fighting Dyslexia

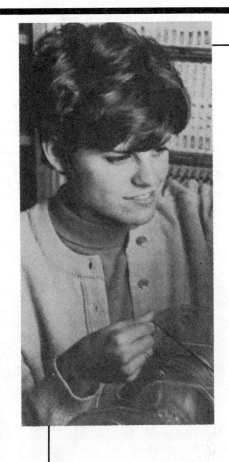

A student who can't read is pursuing an engineering career at Columbia University's School of Engineering and Applied Science, and with the school's blessing.

Kathy Rice, 23, has dyslexia, the inability to link the written word with the spoken word or idea. Oddly enough, however, Kathleen, like many dyslexics, can readily recognize figures and diagrams. Before coming to Columbia, she held jobs at two engineering firms, where she had no trouble reading blueprints or charts. Her job success encouraged her to study engineering. She hopes to complete work for a degree in civil engineering by January, 1977.

An engineering curriculum isn't all charts and blueprints, however, so Kathy Rice had her textbooks taped free by Recordings for the Blind. She avoids courses that demand too much taping. The average math book takes up to 15 four-track tapes and requires up to 60 hours of listening. It's a slow way of acquiring knowledge, but she can read only a few words without becoming exhausted. Some dyslexics do learn to read, but her condition was not diagnosed until she was 13, too late to enter a special reading course for dyslexics.

Before her problem was diagnosed, Kathy Rice was a failure in most subjects. Afterwards, her parents read her books to her and she did so well she became Valedictorian of her high school.

"Fighting Dyslexia," *Science Digest*, Vol. 77 No. 6, June 1975. ©1975 The Hearst Corporation.
"Some Principles of Remedial Instruction For Dyslexia," N. Dale Bryant, Ph.D., *Learning Disorders: Special Report*, No. 2, April 1965.

Teaching Comprehension to the Disabled Reader

CARITA A. CHAPMAN

As Director, Bureau of Reading Improvement, Chicago Board of Education, Chapman is responsible for reading programs in the Chicago Public Schools.

Although the general consensus is that comprehension of the printed word is the acme of what is called "reading," agreement does not exist as to which comprehension skills are most useful to the reader. With older disabled readers, some techniques have emerged as being more successful than others for developing reading comprehension skills. This article presents a framework within which to consider these techniques and suggests classroom approaches.

The students in junior and senior high school who range from nonreaders with such low reading levels that they are unable to function in the classroom, to those retarded a year or two in terms of potential are of crucial concern to educators because: 1) they have difficulty comprehending printed materials at their grade placement; 2) the older they are, the harder it is to correct their problems, and this now represents "a last chance" for severely retarded readers; 3) their time is at a premium for soon they will be adult citizens expecting an opportunity to reap the personal, social, economic, and political benefits accorded to society's literates; and 4) their teachers are primarily subject-matter specialists, unprepared and reluctant to teach students how to read their subject matter.

To provide remediation for these students, it is imperative that teachers weave together the three separate strands of 1) specific reading comprehension skills, 2) materials in the content areas, and 3) methods using all modalities (hearing, seeing, body movement). Combining these strands should be done in the least amount of time but with the greatest amount of structural organization, including only the fundamental components to enable both teacher and student to know exactly "where we're going, how, and with what."

The essential components for developing the reading comprehension skills show three dimensions, like a pillar of bricks. Just as each horizontal layer of bricks can be thought of as intersecting vertical layers, each learning dimension cuts across the others: 1) reading comprehension skills, 2) methods/modality, and 3) materials/content. The intersection of a specific reading skill, a specific content material, and a specific method or modality forms a brick in the pillar. With the three dimensions of the pillar, the teaching/learning bricks can be arranged intuitively from simple to complex, although in practice no specific sequence of teaching-learning need be followed.

Reading comprehension skills are conceived of in three levels. The literal level is the ability to understand ideas and information explicitly stated in the printed material—"reading the lines." The non-literal level requires getting meanings that are implied—"reading between the lines"—or requires personal judgment, evaluation, or innovation—"reading beyond the lines." Finally, functional skills involve selecting and organizing specific information through use of the previous skills.

Each of these comprehension skills can be taught and practiced through use of each of the three modalities of learning—visual, auditory, and kinesthetic. To speed and reinforce learning, it is important to select learning activities to activate multiple modalities at the same time; in other words, "see it, hear it, and say, draw, or write it."

The content to be learned and on which to practice the skills comes from materials in the four major subject areas: literature, social studies, science, and mathematics. At the high school level, use of material required in the regular courses seems logical and practical and helps insure proper transfer of learned skills. However, this does not exclude the use of materials from other sources.

Classroom Techniques

The following section illustrates ways of combining these separate elements into a coherent whole—that is, to provide a synthesis of successful techniques for helping disabled readers develop reading comprehension.

Comprehension begins on the literal level with **sentence comprehension**—the understanding of sentence structures (the way words are used in relationship to each other), which are the "basic building blocks of meaning" (Lefevre, 1964).

Starting with sentences you are sure the learners can understand, have students dictate a group experience story (which is a type of literature). Write it on the chalkboard and have each student write her or his own copy. This activity employs all sensory tracts: hearing the dictated story, reading it while copying, and using muscle movements to copy it.

Using examples from experience stories and from books in different subject areas, discuss the classifications of Actor, Action, Object (Result, Recipient) and show

"Teaching Comprehension To The Disabled Reader," Carita A. Chapman, *Journal of Reading*, Vol. 20 No. 1, October 1976. ©1976 The International Reading Association, Inc.

the similarity of word order in spoken and written sentences. Lefevre has listed four main sentence patterns of which teachers should be aware: noun-verb (noun-verb-adjective and noun-verb-adverb), noun-verb-noun, noun-verb-noun-noun, and noun-linking verb-noun (noun-linking verb-adjective and noun-linking verb-adverb).

Using these patterns to show how sentences are built, have students substitute many words (orally or in writing) that can make sense in the same positions, first with synonyms, later such ones as "The little lady slapped Bob's dog" becoming "The friendly girl loved the boy's pet." Or, use grammatical markers to outline possible sentences and have pupils put words that make sense into the blanks: The _____ _____ _____ _____ a _____ on the _____ .

Here are several other exercises that help students become aware of the meanings we get from understanding word order and word-class relationships: 1) Make meaningful substitutions for words in nonsense sentences; for example, "The iggle oggled the uggle" (attributed to C.C. Fries). 2) Place scrambled sentences in logical order. 3) Identify a word that spoils the meaning of the sentence; for example, "Lefevre has listed four gulp main sentence patterns." 4) Construct a sentence collage with words selected from newspapers and magazines. These exercises, if extended to develop two or three coordinated sentences, can be used when working on the next levels of comprehension.

Progressing to another level of syntactic awareness, help students discover the transformation of active sentences to passive, using again the Actor-Action-Object categories; for example, changing "The girl threw the ball" to "The ball was thrown by the girl."

Teach them to change declarative sentences to interrogatives (Thomas, 1965), using the question words that begin with wh- ("who," "where," and so on). For example, show a sentence with a unit of meaning underlined: "The little boy fell down." Ask the students to imagine that they heard someone mumble that sentence and that they didn't hear the underlined words clearly; what question word would they use to get the speaker to repeat just the unclear words? ("Who?") Show the following patterns:

"Who" ("whom," "whose") or "what" replace nouns
"What kind of," "which," "how many" replace adjectives
"When," "where," "how," "why" replace adverbs
"What" (+ auxiliary, if present) + "do" replace verbs

The interrogative process can be used with sentences the students have already worked on in doing semantic substitutions, transformations from active to passive, or combinations of both.

Since the ability to answer questions about what one has read is still the most objective and frequently used method of demonstrating comprehension, disabled readers need training in the relationship of questions to sentences. The most literal level of sentence comprehension develops through wh-question transformations. These can be practiced on sentences from textbooks.

After answering questions literally, older pupils benefit from seeing how the literal meaning of a sentence can be expanded to develop higher level comprehension through the use of different types of questions. For instance, ask questions such as: "Tell me in your own words how_____? What facts in the sentence tend to support the idea that _____? What does the writer mean by the phrase _____? What will _____ lead to?" These questions develop inference comprehension. Another type is: "The author says that _____ felt _____. Is this a fact or the author's opinion? How do you know? Do you think the author is right?" These questions tend to develop critical reading skills.

Some words in a sentence have more meaning than others. Teaching students to locate the key words in a sentence is a precursor to locating the topic sentence or main idea of a paragraph. Ask the students which words they would use to send a telegram with the information in this sentence: "The baseball game will take place in Yankee Stadium on Tuesday, June 16th at one o'clock." Continue sending "oral telegrams" or underlining important words in written sentences which progress from the simple to more complex.

In conjunction, students can gain an auditory feel for how meaning can be changed by altering intonation patterns in such a simple sentence as "We like bugs." Relate these experiences to the study skill of recognizing typographical aids—boldface and italic type, headings, subheadings—as other ways of stressing important words and phrases. Having students determine which words and phrases should be stressed in sentences helps them develop those aspects of study skills that deal with notetaking and summarizing.

An important but seldom taught and often misunderstood skill is the comprehension of anaphora—the understanding of grammatical substitutes which refer to a preceding word or group of words. Usually anaphora are pronouns, such as "them" in "The stolen papers were important; the FBI tried to buy *them* back." Another frequent one is the use of "does" to avoid repetition of another verb: "Mary dances better than June *does* (*does* replacing *dances*). Using the students' own constructed sentences in addition to those from their textbooks, have them delete the anaphora and put in its place the correct antecedent to determine "if the sentence makes sense." Test their comprehension of the anaphora by asking: "What does _____ mean? What does _____ refer to?"

Intersentence comprehension refers to understanding the structural relationships between sentences in a paragraph. The order in which sentences appear conveys

3. INSTRUCTIONAL TECHNIQUES

information, just as does the order of words within a sentence. Begin by having students discuss the relationship between two contiguous sentences in a paragraph. This exercise might include cause-effect; time of occurence; listing; comparison-contrast; and either-or.

As part of intersentence comprehension, develop the concept of a topic sentence—it is what the paragraph is all about, whereas the comment sentences (often called "details") enlarge upon the statement made by the topic sentence.

Read short paragraphs aloud to students and discuss them, since students need <u>teaching</u> to understand the concept of topic sentences, not just exercise-answering.

Begin by having students select the main idea from multiple choice alternatives. Progress to having the students write their own main ideas of the paragraph. Use pictures of some action and let students generate possible main ideas, explaining why suggestions would be acceptable or not—often they will be too broad, too narrow, inaccurate, or not included in the picture. Be sure to provide practice in finding the topic sentence in different locations within the paragraph, at the beginning, middle,

end, or inferred. Practice in writing titles or headlines for paragraphs is another way of expressing the main idea.

Outlining, often considered a study skill, evolves naturally from understanding the relation of main idea or topic sentence (represented by Roman numerals) to subordinate sentences (represented by letters). Summarizing is another "study skill" which is related to intersentence comprehension. At this point, PQRST [Preview, Question, Read, Summarize, and Test] (Spache and Berg, 1966) can be introduced as a study method for retaining content.

As students work with intersentence relationships in paragraphs, from different subject matter, instances abound for developing inferences and conclusions and making generalizations; making critical judgments and evaluating for bias or relevancy; and creating new ideas as a result of reading. Correlating as many skills as needed to derive meaning from a paragraph tends to help the retarded reader derive more meaning from those passages he does read, instead of waiting until each level has been "mastered" before proceeding to the next. Likewise, work with intersentence relationships acts as a

stimulus to teaching the locational skills for pursuing further information—use of the library card files, encyclopedias, the dictionary, indexes, maps, and globes.

Tune In, Act Out

This is an intensive, condensed, highly interrelated approach to the direct teaching and learning of reading comprehension skills for high school retarded readers. In addition to using the structured program to "turn on" the students so that they will tune us in and act out their learning roles with increased skill, teachers need to:

• Teach only those skills students do not know, skipping those they do know.

• Set immediate, achievable goals with the student.

• Reward every success with clear signs—charts and stars work even at this level!

• Build the students' self-confidence so that they can succeed through earned praise (as one teacher remarked, "You're forever stroking the ego").

• Teach whatever prior skills are needed; assistance should be given whenever word attack or other skills are needed, even while focusing on comprehension skills.

The Creative Response

Cathy Golden

Education Department, Brown University, Providence, Rhode Island

Of the 15 students in the ninth grade reading class, Fred, in particular, is unresponsive and disinterested. He will not read aloud and seldom listens to anyone else read. Occasionally, he attempts to disrupt the class by poking the student next to him, wriggling, and falling off his chair. A firm direction to stop usually halts his acting out behavior but does not increase his ability to concentrate. Although Fred has a normal IQ he has been unsuccessful with academic work and has been referred for psychological and educational evaluation. For the present, a graduate student from a nearby university is working with Fred and four other students in the class and, with help from various teachers and professionals in the community, has developed a plan to increase Fred's performance in the reading class. Although the strategy described below is designed to increase reading performance, the principles used could be adapted for other subject areas.

Performance Objectives

Each student will list the steps necessary to write a book according to goals formulated by the group.

Together, the group will divide the responsibilities necessary to complete the book.

Each student will make, write and read three pages of the book.

Teaching Strategies

The Book Improvement Test, made specifically for this ninth grade reading group, is similar to the Unusual Uses Test developed by Getzels and Jackson and the Product Improvement Test of the Minnesota Test for Creativity, both of which require students to list either changes or uncommon uses for ordinary objects, such as bricks, pencils, paper clips, stuffed animals, and so forth. The test along with some students' responses appears below.

Follow Through

Students responded to the test individually and later shared their responses with the group.

A brainstorming session produced a list of 60 improvements based mostly on appeal to the five senses. From these suggestions the group decided to make a book which describes a sensory experience in which the words feel, smell, or taste according to their meaning. The word *rough* is made from sandpaper letters; the word *soft* is made from letters cut from cotton flannel; the word *chocolate* is made from chocolate bits; the word *warm* is made from tinfoil. Glitter, used frequently for emphasis, produced a visual and tactile effect when the meaning of a word could not be evoked in a literal way.

Fred contributed art work to the book as well as ideas and printed words. Teachers and students, previously unaware of Fred's talent, found much to admire in his illustrations. Fred increased the amount of time spent in working with reading materials and with the group constructed an original work, "Touch Me." Sharing imaginative ideas and working together on the book helped us all to cope better with the repetitiveness of practicing spelling and reading skills.

"The Creative Response," Cathy Golden, *Learning Disabilities Guide*, Vol. 43 No. 7, December 1976. ©1976 Bureau of Business Practice, Inc.

THE BOOK IMPROVEMENT TEST

Below is a picture of an ordinary book. In the spaces provided list the cleverest, most interesting and unusual ways you can think of for changing this book to make it more enjoyable to read and use. Do not worry about how much money the changes will cost. Think only about what would make the book more interesting for you!

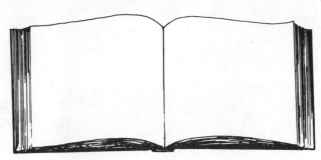

1. Book that would explain everything you don't know.
2. Characters that come out of the book and act as if in a play
3. A book that is big enough to hide in
4. A book about sports that you can go in and play with the characters.
5. A book that has a revolving globe; you spin the globe and push a button and you are where you end up.
6. Silk pages and characters in material costumes
7. Words feel as they mean ⌣ soft as in cotton; words taste as they should ⌣ chocolate
8. When you're talking about food, you can smell and taste the words; food that you can take out, eat and smell.
9. Washable book ⌣ throw it in the washing machine

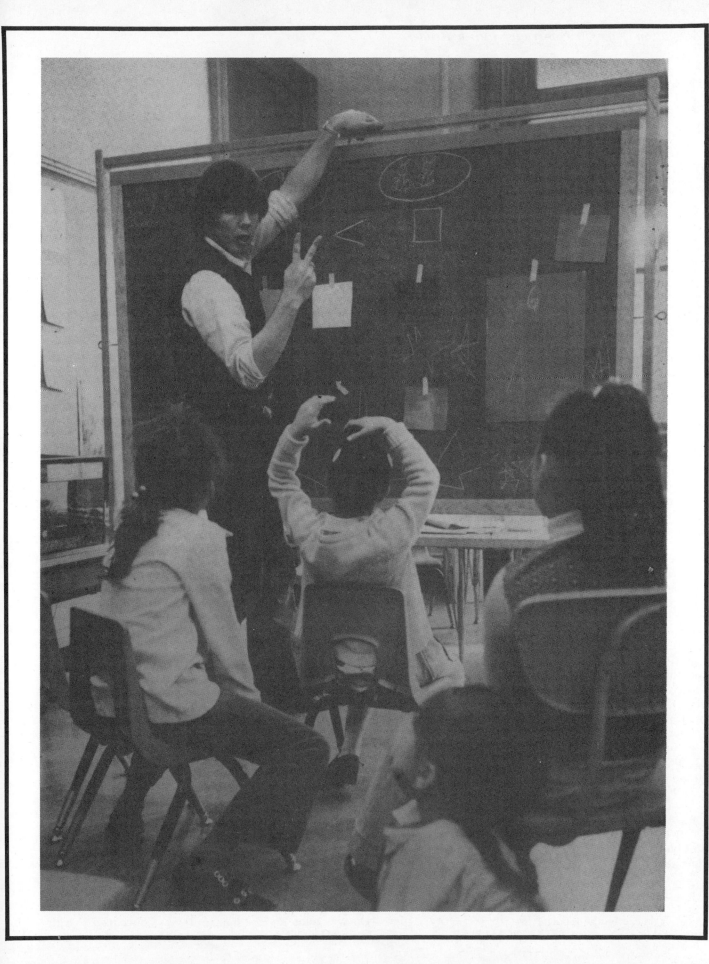

Motivation Turns a Nonreader into a Reader

Thirteen Hours with George

VERNE PETERS

Verne Peters is an instructor of Reading and Language Arts, Parkway North Senior High School, St. Louis, Missouri.

"I don't need to read anything," George said. "I can figure out stuff by myself."

George couldn't read material above second-grade difficulty. But he was promoted to fifth grade anyway. He was 10 years old, happy, healthy, and in the superior range of intelligence. He was not culturally disadvantaged. He had three brothers, a dog, a bicycle, and a workshop in the basement where his father helped him with his favorite hobby—electronics.

George practiced his viola daily, rode his bicycle, swam, and followed the activities of the athletic teams at the university. His younger brothers were learning to read, but George wasn't. He hated books.

I had four weeks to turn this young man on to reading. I was one of a long list of special teachers who had tried to help George. The result was always the same: There was no serious problem which would prevent George from reading except motivation.

Every reading material that was used to motivate him was listed in his file. The diversity was impressive, but each had a readability of first or second grade.

George's mother brought him to the reading center four days a week for four weeks. The Fourth of July and one absence brought our total time together to 13 hours.

I began with nonreading activities. "Let's pretend we are newspaper reporters out to get a story," I said. "You can be the reporter first and take notes as you interview me." George asked good reporter-like questions about my hobbies, my occupation, my home town, and my interests. Examining his notes after he left was a different matter, however. The handwriting was poor, the spelling was poor. Word endings were seldom written, and vowels were often omitted or incorrect. The only positive evaluation I could make was that he had a firm understanding of initial consonants.

George needed to start all over in reading. I had to find something he wanted to read which would challenge him.

The next day I brought in a crossword puzzle. "That's too easy," George said. He was right. He knew all the answers immediately, but didn't know how to spell the words. He would write the initial consonant, then guess at the rest based on the number of squares. My sounding out the syllables didn't help, which meant he had no knowledge of phonics.

The last ten minutes of the hour I read part of a mystery story to George, stopping at an exciting moment to maintain interest for the next day. There was no problem with his memory or comprehension. Each day George paraphrased what I had read the previous day before I began reading the next segment.

The third day was a disaster because I asked George to read. I cut apart a page of cartoons and separated their captions. George was to select the right caption for each picture. He guessed correctly, but refused to read the captions to me. "You can read them yourself," he said.

Together, we wrote a progressive story, but it was not very successful, either. It took too much time. George was a master at diversionary tactics. "Do you want to hear about the hi-fi system I built?" he asked.

Each day I tried to relate reading to electronics in some way. Later, I tried to show George that it was important for him to read about electronics.

A progress chart proved to be a good motivational technique. The chart included behavioral goals as well as reading skills. He scored a point for using time wisely, playing games fairly, wearing his reading glasses, using good reading posture, and listening. Reading skills included analyzing new words, reading orally with expression, using the dictionary, writing legibly, and spelling correctly. A prize was to be awarded for scoring 100 points; a bonus for 150 points.

When the mystery story was completed I brought in a *Mechanics Illustrated* and told George to choose an article for me to read. At first he chose the cover story, which eliminated his having to read the table of contents. Then I read the table of contents to him. George always chose an article on electronics and took the magazine home with him each night.

A Treasure Hunt

One week passed quickly. Most of our reading activities involved games, contests, puzzles, comics, or riddles which disguised the reading skills George was learning. A treasure hunt was George's favorite game. Ten clues which led to the treasure (a sack of his favorite candy) were hidden in the reading center rooms and yard. The rules forbade me to help him, but the dictionary was allowed and was available. I followed George silently, watching him painfully decipher each clue. He liked the hunt so much he planned one for me.

Despite the success of the treasure hunts, I was discouraged with George's progress. I knew that

 "Thirteen Hours With George," Verne Peters, *The Education Digest*, Vol. XL No. 9, May 1975. ©1975 Prakken Publishing reading seldom involved games, contests, or treasure hunts. More often reading was linked to information, study, or plot. I feared that once the prizes were won George would return to his pattern of getting by without reading. I had only seven hours left.

Utilizing a Book on Tape

He was still unwilling to read a book orally until an idea and a stopwatch came to my rescue. George loved to time the contests we had in looking up programs in the *TV Guide* or words in the dictionary.

Using a commercial tape of a book, I bet George that he could read the first chapter in the same time as the voice on the tape. "Aw, it would take me all day to read that much," he said. "I don't think so, George. If you listen carefully to the tape and follow each word in your book as you listen, you'll remember the words. I'm willing to bet you a soda that you can. Even if you can't, you still win the soda. How can you lose?"

"OK, I'll try," he said. George glued his eyes to the book as he listened intently to the tape and clutched the stopwatch in his hand. Then he reset the watch and began reading orally. His reading was fairly accurate because of his good memory. The tape took eight minutes; George took 15. I lost the bet but won a major challenge.

Our last five hours together were spent playing Scrabble and reading *Mechanics Illustrated.* George agreed to read orally for 10 minutes by the stopwatch. He chose articles on updating hi-fi speakers, building an intercom system, building an electric cycle, building a color TV, and on new innovations in electronics of the future. He was familiar with the technical vocabulary, but he could not read it without my helping him analyze the words using phonics. (The articles proved to be tenth-grade readability using the Dale-Chall formula.)

Our last day together was the most satisfying to me in several ways. George had earned more than 200 points on his progress chart, yet he worked harder the last hour than ever before. While playing Scrabble he noticed that I had forgotten to bring the dictionary. "I'll get it," I said. "No," said George, "I don't want to waste any time our last day together." He ran all the way to the library for the dictionary and beat me again at Scrabble.

At the cafeteria, George piled his tray with three drinks, two desserts, the main course, and a salad. I was paying for a lunch at which he could choose anything he wanted to eat and have all the seconds he wanted, as the prize he had selected for earning his 100 points. Over lunch we discussed how neat it would be if he could read *Mechanics Illustrated* without my help. He agreed, and hinted broadly that he could read it if he had his own subscription.

Thirteen hours with George uncovered one important reason for him to read. With the magazine coming into his home each month (his bonus prize), and parents and teachers helping him, I'm confident more reasons will surface.

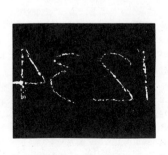

TUTORING EXPERIENCE FOR DISABLED READERS

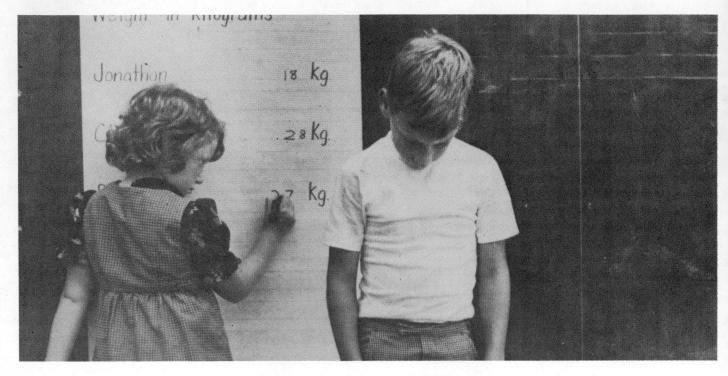

LAWRENCE L. SMITH

Indiana State University, Terre Haute, Indiana

The future prospects of a high school student having great difficulty with reading and writing skills are not very reassuring. With almost every class attended, he meets frustration. He cannot read the text and finds his papers full of red ink because of his inability to spell or express his thoughts. If a school is fortunate enough to have a remedial or corrective reading teacher, some help can be offered to this student. Progress, however, is frequently negligible, and often the high school student is not "turned on" to working on reading skills. He may go through the motions, but his heart is not in the task. Consequently, he does not learn to read and write well, he remains frustrated, and quite possibly will drop out of school.

There is an alternative, however, to most remedial or corrective reading programs offered for secondary students. A special program, presently being used at Indiana State University Laboratory School, should improve the students' attitudes and language arts skills. For years students have been taught to tutor other students, and such programs have met with success; but most of the time an intermediate grade student has been sent to a primary grade to "help" the teacher, and in a few places, high school students have been sent to elementary buildings. Through a program of the latter type, the high school students, as well as the elementary student, should find that his reading skills improve.

Necessary to make this program effective are what I call the "3 T's" of tutoring. They are *training, teaching,* and *translating.*

Training

The high school tutor is scheduled into the reading room approximately fifteen to twenty minutes before the elementary student is due to arrive. This is the time when the reading teacher may train the student for the specific skills to be taught. This activity is extremely important, because, quite possibly, the high school student may not know all the words in the lesson he is to teach, he may need to practice the story that he will read to the student, or he, himself, may need to be taught a skill for teaching word recognition.

Teaching

The elementary student is scheduled to be in the reading room for about thirty minutes, allowing the other ten minutes for a "fun activity" such as playing "Phonic Rummy," working a crossword puzzle with the high school student, working riddles, or reading a story to each other. Games such as these reinforce reading skills as well as establish a working relationship for the elementary student and his tutor.

Translating

After the elementary student has returned to his room, the high school tutor should evaluate his own role and performance with the younger student. Evaluation is a very important part of the high school student's lesson, because this is when he works on his writing skills. Since these students have difficulty expressing their ideas, some beginning guideline questions have been given, and the student keeps a log using these questions. Suggestions for questions are:

"Tutoring Experience for Disabled Readers," Lawrence L. Smith, *Reading Improvement*, Vol. 10, No. 1, Spring 1973.
©1973 Project Innovation.

1. What materials did you use today?
2. Describe at least one successful task accomplished by your student.
3. Do you think your student enjoyed the tasks you asked him to do? Please explain.
4. How do you feel about helping your student with his work today?
5. Did you find any part of the lesson difficult to teach?

When using a program such as this, all language art skills are being developed. The bonus is that many of the high school students feel a great responsibility toward helping the elementary student, and they show great concern for him.

Some examples of responses high school students make are exemplified by their answers to question four of the guide questions.

"He felt like doing his work and I felt like helping him."

"I try to teach him but he play around to much and wouldn't listen."

"He did it real good. He likes SRA, but he didn't like reading that book. I like working with Gary, and he like working with me."

"I like working with Steve very much today. Steve is nice to work with but he has a lot of trouble."

"I like working with Carl, he is a good boy."

"I feel like he always likes his work and tries his hardest."

We are not too forceful with the high school tutor, but offer suggestions to him about his log and urge his teacher to use the log as part of his English requirement. High school students have proved very receptive to this type of program, as well as to suggestions on how a student can improve his spelling or how he can make a sentence more meaningful.

It appears that a tutoring program such as the one suggested can improve the high school student's attitude and language art skills. It is very important that the student have preparation time before teaching, just as the professional teacher would not want to teach a lesson unless prepared. The working time should probably not exceed twenty minutes, with some time left for a "fun activity." Last, but certainly not least, the writing of the log helps the student improve his writing skills, and hopefully, gives him some insight into how he might help himself improve his own reading skills. And of course a program like this helps the remedial reading teacher help more elementary students.

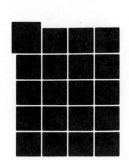

FOCUS...

A New Alphabet

Current reading approaches incorporate changes in the traditional twenty-six letter alphabet. This example illustrates changes which have been made to assure regular correspondence between sound and symbol to eliminate multiple spellings of the same sound. It is considered to be a change in medium and not in methodology.

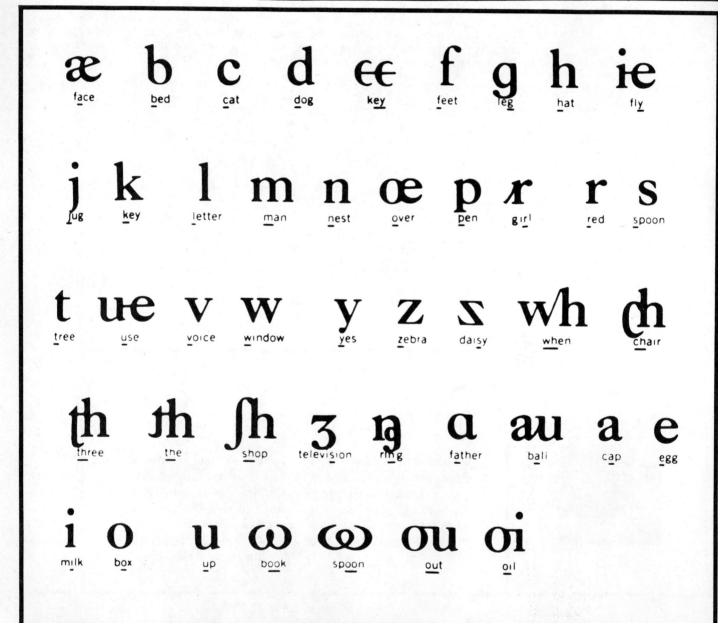

Used with the permission of Initial Teaching Alphabet Publications, Inc.,
6 East 43rd Street, New York, New York 10017.

Handwriting of Mike: 10 years old

TO DAY IST HUTSa
a YIT IS aLO | 0/0/04
NENV||180TO8YN

Handwriting of Allen: 10 years old

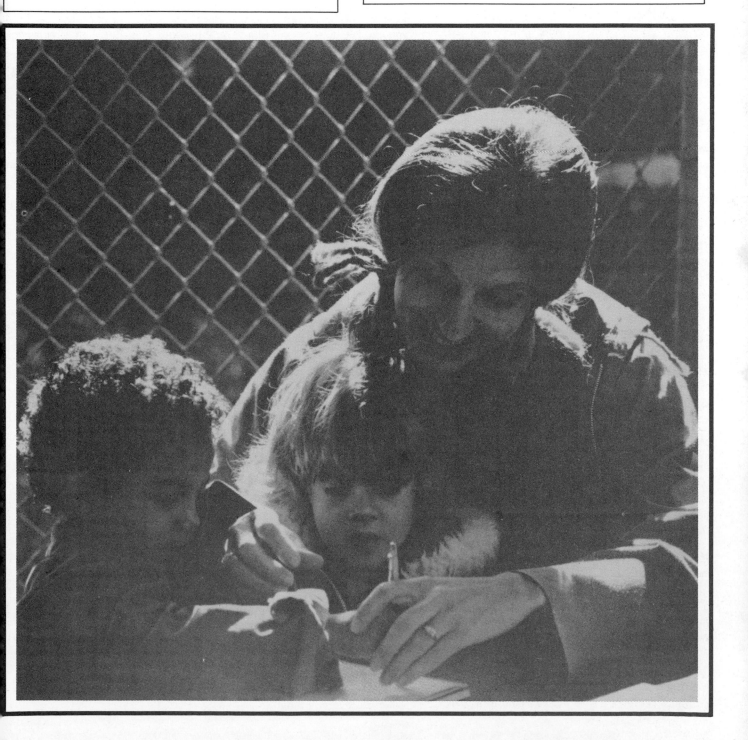

Braille: A Language for Severe Dyslexics

Lois E. McCoy, M.S.

Braille is suggested as an alternative language for the severely learning disabled student; it is a ready-made language and it uses a completely different pathway than that of auditory/visual input. The apparent success using this technique with a 15-year-old girl who could neither read nor write seems to justify consideration of this radical approach to teaching a method of communication to the severe dyslexic. Instruction in Braille began for this girl in September 1973, and within four months she had exceeded her highest previous reading achievement. In June 1974, she began fourth-grade studies in Braille, and a whole new world of information was opened to her through her newly found skills and the Talking Books and tape-recorded information which accompanied her Braille program.

The learning disability syndrome, for the average elementary school teacher, was still a relatively unknown and unrecognized problem in the fall of 1963, when Roslyn entered kindergarten. With the exception of a few interested educators and parents assembling the first formal groups to try to understand the neurologically disabled child, children with such problems received little help or understanding. Ten years later her clearly recognizable symptoms would have been quickly detected, although present techniques could have done little to help her.

My daughter Roslyn may be an atypical example of what is called the learning disabled child, but surely she is a good example of severe dyslexia. While the program presented here would be far too radical for mass use with dyslexic students, it might be the only possible teaching method for a few who have not found success with any previously used technique. This method involves the use of Braille, which is known to be a successful method of written communication for the blind. The Library of Congress Division for the Blind and Physically Handicapped, the American Printing House for the Blind, and the American Foundation for the Blind, Inc., all have stores of material available translated into Braille or recorded as Talking Books. Thus, Braille suggested itself as a ready-made alternative method which might allow the dyslexic child to communicate through a written language system.

Roslyn's school experience had consisted of five years of frustration and failure. She had repeated both first and third grades. The administrators in the school district in California were finally convinced that Roslyn had a problem that was neither psychological nor a matter of slow maturity. Every technique available to her through the public educational systems in California and later in Colorado was explored, as well as private techniques including Doman-Delacato (1968), reading specialists in Los Angeles, Educationally Handicapped classes and Science Research Associates programs. Countless medical specialists and psychologists examined her and tested her, providing diagnoses ranging from mentally retarded to unusually gifted and creative. In spite of a superior range IQ her reading and writing ability did not improve beyond mid-second grade. It was clear that the impairment involved visual sequential order and auditory digit memory storage, as well as a visual focusing problem. Her vision and hearing acuity were normal and health was excellent.

Essentially Roslyn's problem was demonstrated by the following: maximum auditory memory of four digits; poor visual digit memory; hazy time concept; continued reversals of letters and numbers beyond age eight; confusion of right/left, East/West, across the street/next door, yesterday/tomorrow; poor/fine motor coordination; EEG -- borderline brain damage of very questionable significance; poor hand/eye coordination; low WISC/Verbal

"Braille: A Language For Severe Dyslexics," Lois E. McCoy, M.S., *Journal of Learning Disabilities*, Vol. 8 No. 5, May 1975. °1975 The Professional Press, Inc.

scores; Auditory Discrimination test: quiet-condition — below 50th percentile, noise-condition — above 70th percentile; and mixed hand and eye dominance.

Her strengths are seen in a superior auditory comprehension memory (equal to a visual photographic memory); no apparent limit to her auditory attention span; excellent gross motor coordination — skiing, ice skating, etc. She also exhibits superior tactile ability; musical and artistic talent (original and non-conformist); well developed abilities of logic and deductive reasoning; high WISC/Performance scores; Raven scores; spring 1971, 59 of 60 correct: fall 1974, 59 to 60 correct. In addition to these strengths she has a tremendous ability to maintain a happy, hopeful approach to life.

It seemed to me that one more neuro-pathway needed to be considered — that of touch — but more than four years passed before an educational system could be found that was willing to invest the time and money in a method that had not to our knowledge been seriously considered before.

Wyburn (1960) states with regard to touch receptors: "Stimulus strength is indicated not only by the greater frequency of discharge of the receptors, but by spreading to other receptors so that there will be a greater volume of impulse input into the central nervous system." As part of an undergraduate class in human neurology, I had spent many extra hours studying the pathways of visual, auditory and touch sensory input. Because of the complex "crossing-over" mechanisms involved in visual and auditory pathways, and because both the visual and auditory pathways involve similar reverberating circuit links within the cerebellum (Snider 1958), it occurred to me that perhaps touch could be an alternative path to learning. Following complex analyses beyond the scope of the present paper, it seemed reasonable to seriously consider the use of Braille. If Roslyn's problem involved some kind of brain malfunction, it seemed unlikely that the quite different pathway of touch would be impaired. While this hypothesis may be partly true, her progress in reading Braille may also be due to an increase in receptors receiving stimulus as seen in her own form of adaptation of the Braille method. For example, Roslyn has greater success in reading and comprehension by combining vision with touch. As she explains, "Using touch alone is slow, my eyes don't always tell the truth so I can't just read the symbols, but I can get the best of both when I use my fingers and eyes together."

Donald G. Doehring's recent impressive study (1973, pp. 41-42) lends further support to my theory that of his 109 measures used to statistically compare normal readers with retarded readers, the reading retardation group showed a significant superiority to the normal reading group on five measures, four of which were tests of tactile ability (one at .001 level and three at .05 level). This finding seems even more significant in light of the present paper.

In the fall of 1973, Mrs. Evelyn C. Whitehead, itinerant teacher of the blind and partially sighted students for Boulder Valley School District in Boulder, Colorado, began teaching her first full-sighted student. Whitehead was also a specialist in remedial reading. She proceeded to work with Roslyn one hour a day throughout the school year first to determine whether the pathway from Roslyn's sense of touch was normal, and then to find out if this girl who had never been able to read the printed word with any measure of success could learn this new and very difficult language. Her Braille training during the past 10 months has included the following general steps: (1) Braille prereading activities — Touch and Tell. (2) Braille alphabet study. (3) Preprimer. (4) Dr. Seuss books and 220 Dolch Basic Words. She maintained a record box of all the words she knew. A record was kept of her progress and usual remedial reading techniques were employed. (5) An attempt was made at writing compositions, but due to the total lack of language skills beyond third grade, this was abandoned for the present. (6) Auditory discrimination in depth for phonetic development, a method which enabled her to learn sounds by how they are placed in the mouth. She learned to associate each group of sounds with a certain action within her mouth. This resulted in an auditory/kinesthetic correlation which proved quite successful. (7) Memorization work in acquiring the necessary 200+ contractions which are part of Grade 2 Braille.*

On June 3, 1974, 15-year-old Roslyn called home and said, "I have a big surprise for you! I have just passed all my tests and have completed all the requirements for third grade!" This was indeed the happiest news in many years. Her phenomenal ability to learn by this method was evident from the first week. Her teacher often remarked that Roslyn's sense of touch was "the most sensitive of any child I have ever taught." Her progress was not without problems, but happily most of these were the same problems that "normal" blind chil-

3. INSTRUCTIONAL TECHNIQUES

dren encounter when they are first learning Braille. At the end of two months Roslyn had progressed beyond a point that would take the average sighted person six months to attain when they first learn Braille. Through her sense of touch she was now able to store and retrieve the Braille symbols for words.

One advantage of the Braille treatment over Talking Books or Tapes is that written communication can emerge — at times demanding the distinction among and at other times the unification of several learning systems. In time, Roslyn was able to construct her own short compositions on the Perkins Brailler, which was the first time she had ever been able to communicate her inner thoughts in writing. She began to sound out words phonetically — a concept she had understood visually, but due to her inability to perceive the proper direction of the word she was studying, was never able to perform successfully. Now under her fingers the words "stay put" and she has little trouble putting the sounds together. In response to her rapid progress, her Braille lessons were increased from five to seven hours a week, and she read until her fingers tingled.

The Library of Congress Division For The Blind and Physically Handicapped has supplied Roslyn with a Talking Book machine and she is kept well supplied with recorded books. A whole new world has opened up to her as she listens to the stories she has always wanted to hear. The lives and work of famous people like John F. Kennedy and Jane Addams fill her hungry mind. She is beginning to find it difficult to find others as aware of historical figures as she is becoming. She is shocked, for example, when she finds that no one seems to know that Franklin D. Roosevelt staked his career on Jane Addam's ideas during his first term as President. "Can you imagine," she states with great indignation, "Roosevelt got credit for all the great things that Jane Addams did and thought of! *She* was responsible for the Child Labor Law, and . . ." It is not unusual for her to stay up all night listening to a book she just can't put down, so to speak. Her favorite subjects are, at this time, history and social studies, the two classes she has never been permitted to attend.

Grade 1 Braille is a one-to-one direct correlation between the alphabetical letters and Braille symbols, which is seldom used. Grade 2 Braille combines the one-to-one correlation of Grade 1 Braille with more than 200 short form symbols for words and word groups. Grade 3 Braille is a shorthand form of Braille which is very difficult and seldom used.

It is anticipated that it will take at least a year, via the Talking Books, to begin to fill in the large gaps in her academic knowledge. Her teacher says, "Her gaps are so great and scattered that I just don't know where to begin." Possibly as the body sometimes craves the food it needs most, Roslyn will be naturally attracted to the subjects she needs most. At least for the present she is allowed freedom to choose whatever books she cares to read. Her retention ability for concepts has always been excellent, which is a great advantage in her being able to assimilate large quantities of knowledge in a short span of time.

Seven months after beginning her Braille study, Roslyn began to become acutely aware of her own pronunciation errors and remarked on how often others mispronounce certain words. This was a new skill that was probably beginning to develop as a result of her being able to perceive the total structure of words and relate that structure to sounds. Earlier attempts to correct her rather "careless" speech had only negative results. Other errors, such as "I don't got it," were very common before Braille training: yet these types of errors seldom occurred after the sixth month. Previous speech problems included use of pronouns in place of nouns, poor and incomplete sentence structure, slurring word endings, and sometimes a mixing of phonetic groups within a word. In spite of these problems she would seldom use a simple word to express herself if she knew a complex word that meant the same thing.

One of the most serious problems at this point in Roslyn's development is her need for constant review. While forgetfulness has been a problem in more areas than simply the academic environment, it is unclear whether this is due to some cerebral malfunction, or to habitual carelessness. Most of the material and concepts she is reading have been previously covered in various ways during her academic experience, though often little understood. As totally new material is increasingly encountered — new spelling words, for example — this problem could prevent the successful acquisition of written communication language skills.

While blind children are able to begin Braille in elementary school, reading a hundred or more books at each level as they move up the educational ladder, the older child cannot tolerate the boredom of the juvenile subjects. Material for the blind, both written and recorded, is for the most part aimed at two extremes of interest, the very young and the aged. Thus, one of the most difficult challenges in program planning is the unavailability of enough material in Braille which combines high interest subjects with low vocabulary levels. Fortunately, Roslyn finds mysteries and fantasy stories interesting, and she will be reading many books from the Morgan Bay Mysteries series (Rambeau 1969) this summer. She will be working essentially on her own, reading as many books in Braille as possible, completing at least one unit a week in her fourth grade speller, and listening to Talking Books.

The techniques suggested here are not yet for group remediation but are applicable on a one-to-one tutorial basis. Roslyn's teacher, who was not only a Braille specialist but also trained in remedial reading, is a rare professional in the field today. This article may suggest the feasibility of training others who could function in both areas and provide new hope for the dyslexic child.

The most serious interference to Roslyn's progress this past year has been due to psychosocial problems related to self-identity, hopelessness, and peer group acceptance. Many of these problems may be the result of her isolation during the past six years from normal peer group interactions. This was due in part to the California policy and attitude toward children in educationally handicapped classes and to the relative inability of the average intermediate level class method to adjust to "different" ways of learning. While great advances are being made in recognizing, understanding, and helping the elementary level learning disabled student, the intermediate and high school level student continues to flounder in an academic desert where support or even empathy is still almost nonexistent. One simple way to alleviate part of the problem would be to de-emphasize the written communication requirements which eliminate most of these students, one way or another, from academic classes. Many of these students become progressively truant; they "turn on" to the drug and alcohol culture groups who accept them as they are, and eventually they drop out of school. Too often no one really notices that they are missing, or cares to ask why.

Roslyn's outlook for the coming year is hopeful, but with understandable reservations. She faces the adjustment to her sixth new school in three years within the same school district, the possible loss of her Braille teacher, the possible acceptance or rejection from new teachers and students, the whole scene of "put-down" when she must say, "Here I am, I want to learn, but I can't read or write." — *Institute for Behavioral Genetics, University of Colorado, Boulder, Colo. 80302.*

REFERENCES
Doehring, D.G.: Patterns of Impairment in Specific Reading Disability. Indiana Univ. Press 1968, reprinted by McGill Univ. Printing Service, 1973.
Doman-Delacato treatment of neurologically handicapped children. Summary statement approved by the Amer. Acad. of Neurol., Pediatrics and others. Develop. Med. Child Neurol., 1968, 10, 243-246.
Rambeau, J., and Runeau, N.: The Mystery of Morgan Castle. San Francisco, Calif., Harr Wagner Publ., 1962. Reprinted by the Amer. Printing House for the Blind, Louisville, Ky.
Snider, R.S.: The cerebellum. Sci. Amer., Aug. 1958.
Wyburn, G.M.: The Nervous System. New York: Academic Press, 1960.

ACKNOWLEDGMENTS
We are indebted to Evelyn Whitehead, whose faith in a new idea, expert teaching techniques, consistent encouragement, and hard work made all this possible. Special thanks to Sandy Singer, Institute of Behavior Genetics, University of Columbia, for her technical assistance and help with my own dyslexia. This research was supported by NIMH Grant #11167.

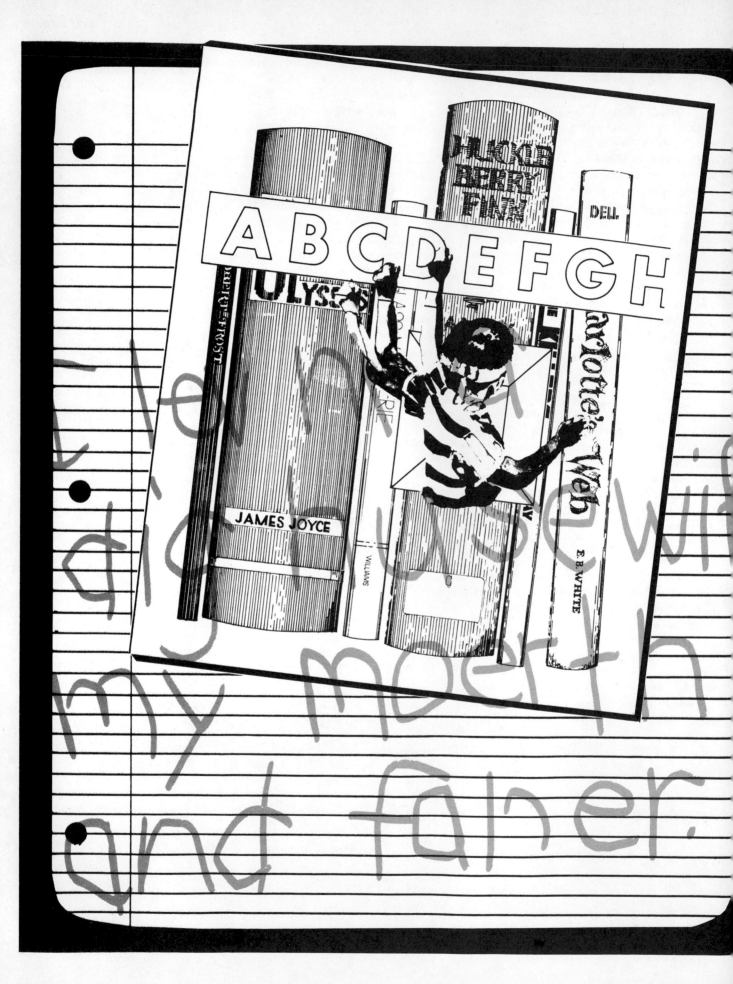

Emerging Concepts

It has been noted that many different methods, techniques, materials, and suspected causes have been studied and examined regarding children with dyslexia. We know that the medical field concentrates its efforts to the area of etiology and that educators relate the disorder to a variety of causes, including inappropriate instruction and poor teaching methods. But what of the very latest concepts? Do they conclude or continue to polarize?

The basal reading series has become the mainstay of reading instruction for the exceptional child, utilizing phonic-based or linguistic-based approaches. The language experience approach utilizes oral and written expression of children, since reading is thought to be a by-product of thinking or oral expression. Other forms of instruction utilize workbooks of programmed reading, or phoneme-grapheme linguistics, which combines oral language with the process of reading skill acquisition.

The most controversial approach has been in phonics. Isolated letter sounds are synthesized and blended into words. Whole new alphabets have been designed to include changes in the traditional twenty-six letter alphabet, which assures a constant correspondence between sound and symbol to eliminate multiple spellings of the same sound. Individualized reading programs allow the child to set his own pace of learning. Multisensory reading approaches attempt to develop reading skills through auditory, visual, tactile and kinesthetic stimulation, while the neurological impress method offers a system where unison reading between the teacher and student is encouraged and the child slides his finger along the line following the words which are being spoken.

None of these approaches can or should be considered a panacea. The problems are so specialized for the dyslexic child, that the future research of diagnosticians and teachers alone holds the most vital key of self-help for the child who cannot read.

IF JOHNNY CAN'T READ, CAN HE COMPUTE?

Edna Warncke
Ball State University, Muncie, Indiana
Byron Callaway
University of Georgia, Athens, Georgia 30602

This investigation was an attempt to determine whether there is a relationship between arithmetic computational ability and reading ability for pupils with normal intelligence who have difficulty in reading. Children, grades two, three and four were administered the WISC, the Fundamentals Section of the California Arithmetic Test and an informal reading inventory. Mean scores were obtained for each grade level for each variable. Pearson product moment correlations were computed to determine if a relationship existed between subject's ability to read and to do fundamental computation. These correlations were not significant. Correlations between grade placement and arithmetic were higher than correlations between reading and arithmetic.

Research which relates reading and arithmetic tends to indicate that poor readers have poor problem solving ability in arithmetic. A number of reports (1) (3) (4) have been published dealing with this relationship. They conclude the importance of teaching reading skills as they relate to mathematics. Generally these studies report high correlations between pupil ability to solve verbal arithmetic problems and pupil ability to comprehend in reading. Authors' chief recommendation for the correction of this problem is for teachers to give special instruction in vocabulary development in the area of mathematics as well as special instruction in how to read mathematical material. If pupils understand what they read, the research infers that they will probably be able to do well in arithmetic problem solving.

What about ability to compute? Is there a relationship between ability to read and ability to do arithmetic computation? What expectation should teachers of poor readers have relative to pupils' ability to compute, if pupils have normal intelligence? Much of the arithmetic encountered by elementary children depends largely on their computational

ability, therefore it would seem worthwhile to investigate the relationship between reading and computational ability.

This investigation was designed to attempt to determine whether there is a relationship between arithmetic computational ability and reading ability for pupils with normal intelligence who have difficulty in reading. Subjects for this investigation were all second, third, and fourth grade referrals to the University of Georgia Reading Clinic between October 1969 and August 1971 provided their IQ was determined to be at least 90. The 75 subjects were: 25 second graders; 25 third graders; and 25 fourth graders. These pupils had been referred to the clinic because of reading difficulty, from all areas of the state of Georgia, representing socio-economic levels from low to high.

All tests were administered to the subjects by the regular clinic personnel. For the purposes of this investigation, the reading level of the subjects was determined by the grade placement yielded on the Informal Reading Inventory (IRI) used in the clinic. This inventory yields reading levels according to the usual basal reader notations, i.e., preprimer,

"If Johnny Can't Read, Can He Compute?" Edna Warncke, Bryon Callaway, *Reading Improvement*, Vol. 10 No. 3, Winter 1973. ©1973 Project Innovation.

primer, first reader, 2^1, 2^2, etc. These notations were converted for purposes of statistical analysis to 1.3, 1.5, 1.7, 2.3, 2.7, etc., respectively. The California *Arithmetic Test,* Form W, was used to determine the fundamental arithmetic ability of the subjects. The test includes addition, subtraction, multiplication, and division. It is published at various grade levels and results reported herein were obtained from the grade level test which was appropriate for the pupil being tested. These included Form W for: Grades 1-2; Grades H2-3-L4; and Grades 4-5-6. Most of the subjects were tested with the H2-3-L4 test, but occasionally the subject was a beginning second grader or a completing fourth grader requiring the use of one of the other two levels of the test. All subjects were also given the Wechsler Intelligence Scale for Children (WISC).

The second grade subjects ranged in grade placement from 2.4 to 2.9 with a mean grade placement of 2.7. Their IRI placement ranged from 1.3 (preprimer) to 2.3 (first half of second grade) with a mean grade placement on the IRI of 1.6. Mean age for the subjects was 7.8 with a mean IQ on the WISC of 108, ranging from 91 to 125. On the fundamentals only section of the arithmetic test, second grade subjects ranged in scores from 1.2 to 4.0 with a mean score of 2.5.

The third grade subjects ranged in grade placement from 3.1 to 3.9 with a mean grade placement of 3.6. Their IRI scores ranged from 1.3 to 3.3 with a mean IRI score of 1.8. Average age of these subjects was 8.6 with mean IQ at 105 ranging from 91 to 129. On the fundamentals only section of the arithmetic test, third grade subjects scored from 1.5 to 4.9 with a mean score of 3.6.

A look at the descriptive data pertaining to the fourth grade subjects reveals that their mean grade placement was 4.5, covering the complete grade level range. Their IRI scores ranged from 1.3 to 3.7 with the mean grade placement according to the IRI falling at 2.3. On arithmetic, the fourth grade mean score was 4.2, ranging from 2.9 to 5.2. These

subjects averaged 9.3 years of age and had a mean IQ score of 102, ranging from 91 to 120.

Pearson product moment correlation coefficients were computed to determine if a relationship existed between the subjects ability to read, as determined by the IRI and his ability to do the fundamental computations necessary for arithmetic, as determined by the *California Arithmetic Test.* A second group of correlations were computed to determine the relationship between the actual grade placement of the subjects, and their performance on the arithmetic. Additional correlations were computed to determine the relationship between the IRI and grade placement and the IRI and the WISC.

The purpose of this investigation was to determine if a relationship existed between the reading ability and the computational ability of these pupils. At the second grade level, the correlation between the IRI and arithmetic was .33. This would indicate a non-significant relationship between the grade placement of the subjects on reading and their ability to compute in arithmetic. At the third grade level, the correlation between the IRI and arithmetic was .0018; at the fourth grade level it was .0010. At both the third and fourth grade levels, this investigation would indicate that there is no appreciable relationship between the performance of these subjects on the Informal Reading Inventory and the Fundamentals section of the *California Arithmetic Test.*

When correlations were computed between the actual grade placement of these subjects and their arithmetic placement, the following correlations were found: second grade .39; third grade .76; fourth grade .68. Correlations between grade placement and arithmetic were much higher than between reading and arithmetic.

All three groups had no appreciable correlations between IRI and grade placement, but correlations between the IRI and the WISC ranged between .51 and .59. This would seem to indicate that there is a closer relationship be-

TABLE 1

Mean Scores for Each Grade Level Relative to Each Variable

	Grade Placement	Age	IRI	Arithmetic	WISC
Grade 2	2.7	7.8	1.6	2.5	108
Grade 3	3.6	8.6	1.8	3.6	105
Grade 4	4.5	9.3	2.3	4.2	102

TABLE 2

Correlations for Paired Variables at
Second, Third, and Fourth Grades

	Arithmetic and IRI	Arithmetic and Grade Placement	IRI and Grade Placement	IRI and WISC
Grade 2	.33	.39	.05	.51
Grade 3	.0018	.76	.03	.56
Grade 4	.0010	.68	.02	.59

tween the IRI placement and intelligence than there is between IRI and grade placement. Although this relationship seems highly unlikely, the explanation relates to the subjects used and would have no generalization validity. These subjects were, by design, of average intelligence and poor reading ability, therefore, reasonably high correlations between these variables would be expected.

As teachers work with problem readers in their classrooms, this investigation would indicate that they might expect their pupils to work fairly close to grade level on computationally based arithmetic, even though they may be one or more grade levels below grade placement in reading. As students reach the intermediate grade levels where arithmetic becomes more dependent upon reading for the solution of verbal problems, earlier research indicates that teachers need to take particular care to help the pupils with the reading aspects of the arithmetic.

Care should be exercised on the part of the reader of this report, not to over-generalize from this investigation. However, cautious generalizations seem feasible since these subjects with reading difficulty, though not randomly selected, did come from a statewide geographic area. One might conclude that although researchers indicate that there is a relationship between reading and arithmetic computational ability at the second, third, and fourth grade levels. If Johnny can't read, he may be able to compute! Teachers—don't sell him short on all counts if he happens to be short in reading!

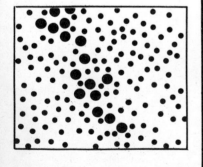

Developmental Dyslexia:

Two Right Hemispheres and None Left

Sandra F. Witelson

Department of Psychiatry, Chedoke
Hospitals, McMaster University,
Hamilton, Ontario, Canada L8N 3L6

Developmental dyslexia, or specific reading disability, refers to the clinical syndrome of difficulty in reading in intellectually, emotionally, and medically normal individuals. Such a deficit is particularly incapacitating in modern, highly literate societies and frequently results in secondary behavioral and emotional difficulties. Estimates of the incidence of the disorder are as high as 5 percent of school-age children, which makes it a prevalent as well as a serious disorder (1).

Numerous etiological hypotheses of dyslexia have implicated various neurological, social, and educational factors (2). None, however, has received strong or consistent support. One long-standing neural hypothesis, originally suggested by Orton (3), implicates abnormal cerebral dominance or functional asymmetry of the hemispheres. Testing this hypothesis has become possible only within the last decade with the development of a number of experimental techniques; for example, tasks requiring the perception of lateralized stimuli allow inferences about hemisphere specialization in nonbrain-damaged individuals (4, 5). Numerous studies using these techniques, particularly dichotic (auditory) stimulation (6) and, to a lesser extent, tachistoscopic stimulation in the lateral visual fields (7),

have been reported with variously defined groups of poor readers. All these studies used linguistic stimuli and addressed themselves to the question of whether the left hemisphere is specialized for linguistic processing in such children; the implicit assumption has been that specialization of the left hemisphere is impaired in dyslexia. This assumption probably arose from the well-established clinical knowledge that acquired alexia or dyslexia is usually associated with lesions in the left (speech dominant) hemisphere (8) and from the fact that reading has traditionally been conceptualized as a language skill. The results of these studies (6, 7) have consistently indicated right-ear and right-visual-field superiorities and, by inference, specialization of the left hemisphere for linguistic processing in poor readers, as is the case in normal individuals. However, in spite of the data, many of these reports contain unfounded suggestions of a lack of, or less strong, specialization of the left hemisphere in dyslexia.

In contrast, I have investigated (i) specialization of the right hemisphere for spatial processing, (ii) specialization of the left hemisphere for linguistic processing, and (iii) the relative participation of the two hemispheres on a task that requires the specialized functions of

both. Performance on the last task may be particularly illuminating for, like reading, it involves both types of cognitive processing (9).

The results indicate that in dyslexics, spatial functions are represented in both hemispheres in contrast to the specialization of the right hemisphere in normal children. In addition, and consistent with the previous studies, dyslexics have the typical pattern of left-hemisphere representation of linguistic functions. Although the left hemisphere may mediate the typical cognitive functions, the results suggest that left-hemisphere processing may be deficient in dyslexics. These two possible neural correlates may result in a cognitive pattern of deficits and biases in dyslexia; specifically, a deficiency in the linguistic, sequential, analytic cognitive mode of information processing, and an intact or even overdeveloped use of the spatial, parallel, holistic mode.

A group of 85 right-handed boys (6 to 14 years of age, $\overline{X} = 10.6$), selected as cases of developmental dyslexia on the basis of extensive pediatric, psychiatric, and clinical psychological assessments, were given a battery of four tests considered to reflect hemisphere specialization. Two tests are considered to be indices of right-hemisphere specialization for spatial processing: (i) "dichhaptic stimulation" with meaningless shapes, a relatively new task, in which two different shapes are simultaneously presented one to each hand, to be perceived by active touch alone (5, 10), and (ii) a tachistoscopic task, adapted from the test procedures originally developed with adults, in which pairs of identical or different figures of people were presented in either the right or left visual half-field and had to be identified as "same" or "different." Specialization of the left hemisphere for linguistic processing was assessed with a typical dichotic stimulation test that used free recall of series of pairs of digits. The final test involved dichhaptic presentation of letters that were to be named by the subject (5). The performance of the dyslexic group on these tests was compared to that of a group of 156 normal, right-handed boys who were matched for age ($\overline{X} = 10.5$ years) and socioeconomic class, who had no history of academic or behavioral difficulty, and who obtained age-appropriate scores on reading and spelling achievement tests.

On the dichhaptic shapes test, the dyslexic group showed no difference in accuracy in recognizing shapes presented to their left and right hands ($\overline{X} = 5.1$ and 5.5, respectively, $t = 1.43$, d.f. $= 61$), in contrast to the normal group, who obtained higher left- than right-hand scores ($\overline{X} = 5.4$ and 4.6, $t = 3.82$, d.f. $= 99$, $P < .001$). Greater left-hand accuracy in the normal group is considered to reflect greater participation of the right hemisphere on this spatial task (5, 10). The lack of hand asymmetry in the dyslexic group suggests, instead, bilateral processing of spatial functions.

This interpretation is corroborated by the results of the visual test of right-hemisphere specialization. The dyslexic group showed no difference in accuracy in the perception of human figures presented in the left and right visual fields ($\overline{X} = 5.8$ and 5.6, respectively, $t = 0.96$, d.f. $= 81$). In contrast, the normal group showed greater accuracy for stimuli presented in the left field ($\overline{X} = 6.0$ and 5.5, $t = 2.28$, d.f. $= 84$, $P < .05$) and, by inference, right-hemisphere specialization for this task. Although the dyslexic and normal groups differed in the pattern of perceptual asymmetry on both the tactual and visual spatial tests, the groups did not differ in total accuracy for either test (tactual test: $\overline{X} = 10.5$ and 10.0; visual test: $\overline{X} = 11.3$ and 11.5, respectively).

On the dichotic test, both groups demonstrated better recall for digits presented to the right than to the left ear. (For the normal group, $\overline{X} = 46.0$ and 42.1, $t = 7.32$, d.f. $= 155$, $P < .001$; for the dyslexic group, $\overline{X} = 41.1$ and 35.6, $t = 5.15$, d.f. $= 84$, $P < .001$). These results suggest that the left hemisphere is specialized for linguistic functions in both dyslexic and normal boys. However, total accuracy of the dyslexics was lower than that of the normal group ($\overline{X} = 76.7$ and 88.2; $t = 8.17$, d.f. $= 239$, $P < .0001$). Such impaired overall performance on this task is similar to that observed for groups of individuals with known dysfunction in the left temporal lobe (11); this performance suggests the possibility of dysfunction in the left hemisphere of dyslexics.

On the dichhaptic letters test, the normal group showed only a tendency toward naming more right- than left-hand letters ($\overline{X} = 6.8$ and 5.6, $t = 1.67$, d.f. $= 27$, $P \doteq .10$), whereas the dyslexic group named significantly more left- than right-hand letters ($\overline{X} = 7.7$ and 6.8, $t = 2.45$, d.f. $= 54$, $P < .02$). There was no difference in total accuracy between the groups ($\overline{X} = 12.5$ and 14.6, respectively, $t = 1.53$, d.f. $= 81$). Both spatial and linguistic processing are considered necessary in this task (5), and, consequently, it may allow the manifestation of individual differences in the relative use of the two cognitive strategies. In dyslexics the left hemisphere appears to be the main linguistic processor. The necessity for it to process the linguistic requirements of this task, albeit minimal, particularly if, as I have suggested, it has a limited capacity to do so, may force the spatial processing in this case to be mediated predominantly by the right hemisphere. Furthermore, the actual superiority for left-hand letters exhibited by the dyslexics may reflect a predominance of right-hemisphere functioning and of spatial cognitive processing on this task. These procedures and some of these results are discussed in greater detail elsewhere (12).

The issue arises as to the possible relationships of the hypothesized bilateral neural representation of spatial processing in dyslexics to (i) their cognitive processing and (ii) their reading difficulty. The available evidence indicates that bilateral representation of a cognitive function that is usually lateralized is not necessarily associated with diminished ability (13, 14). Similarly, in this report, in which bilateral spatial representation is hypothesized for dyslexics, there is no

evidence that their spatial processing is deficient. Their mean scaled score on the Wechsler Intelligence Scale for Children (WISC) Block Design subtest was 11.3, which indicates at least average ability and is not different from that of 11.9 for the normal group ($t = 1.30$, d.f. $= 239$). The dyslexic group's mean WISC Performance Intelligence Quotient (IQ), reflecting various aspects of visuospatial processing, was 107, within the average range, and was greater than their Verbal IQ of 97.4 ($t = 5.49$, d.f. $= 84$, $P < .001$). Furthermore, they were as accurate on the two lateral perception tests involving spatial processing as the normal group. The conclusion that at least most dyslexics have normal or better visuospatial perception was previously drawn by Benton (15), in contrast to widespread belief to the contrary, and is further corroborated by a growing body of data (16).

Bilateral representation of a cognitive process could, however, affect cognition by overloading one hemisphere and interfering with those functions "native" to it. Levy (13) observed that some left-handed individuals have lower spatial than verbal ability and suggested, in a vein similar to that of Lashley concerning the neural localization of function (17), that this may be due to the higher incidence of bilateral representation of language in sinistrals and the resultant interference with the right hemisphere's processing of spatial information. In the case of dyslexics, bilateral representation of spatial functions could overload the left hemisphere and interfere or be incompatible with its specialized role in sequential, linguistic processing. Interference with left-hemisphere processing should lead to poor performance on linguistic tasks, as was observed in the present study: the dyslexic group was impaired in overall performance on the verbal dichotic test; the Verbal IQ was significantly lower than the Performance IQ; and the mean scaled score on the WISC Vocabulary subtest was 10.2, which is lower than the normal group's score of 11.4 ($t = 3.44$, d.f. $= 239$, $P < .001$). The hypothesis of deficient left-hemisphere processing is further supported by the results of many studies which indicate that dyslexics show deficits specifically on cognitive tasks that require sequential processing or verbal encoding of information (18), considered to be left-hemisphere functions. Dysfunction per se in the left hemisphere was directly suggested on the basis of the similarity of impaired recall of dichotic stimulation in dyslexics and in patients with known dysfunction in the left temporal lobe.

Deficiency in linguistic, sequential, analytic processing, whether resulting from interference or dysfunction per se in the left hemisphere, could lead to predominant use, wherever possible, of the other cognitive mode, the spatial, parallel, holistic mode, with which dyslexics appear to have no difficulty. The dyslexic group's performance on the dual processing task of dichhaptic letters supports such speculation. In contrast to normal boys, they showed a significant left-hand superiority and, by inference, greater right-hemisphere participation and greater use of spatial, holistic processing. This finding may have relevance for the reading process in dyslexics, since reading also involves dual cognitive processing. In reading, dyslexics may predominantly use a spatial, holistic cognitive strategy and ignore or ineffectively use a phonetic, analytic strategy; such a cognitive strategy bias may be a disadvantage in learning to read. There is evidence compatible with these suggestions. Poor readers appear to make phonetic rather than optical errors (19). Children with marked difficulty in learning to read English readily learned to read (that is, associate with English words) Chinese logographs (20), which depend on visual, holistic processing and not on phonetic, analytic decoding. However, studies with normal children suggest that phonetic encoding facilitates reading progress (21). From the opposite perspective, poor spatial ability is not necessarily associated with reading difficulty. Individuals with Turner's syndrome (XO karyotype) have well-documented specific deficits in spatial processing but have normal reading ability [reported for the English language, which is phonetically coded (22)]. Females, who are generally less proficient on spatial tasks than most men (23), have a much lower incidence of reading difficulty (1). It has not yet been determined whether reverse obser-

vations hold for the reading of ideographic languages.

Thus, at the neural level, developmental dyslexia may be associated with bilateral processing of spatial functions and with deficient left-hemisphere processing of linguistic functions. The left hemisphere may not execute its specialized functions well, but it is not necessarily inactive or ineffectual; it may engage in right-hemisphere types of cognitive processing. This raises the possibility that in dyslexics the left hemisphere does not have focal but, instead, has the right-hemisphere type of diffuse neural organization in terms of Semmes' (24) hypothesis of the nature of hemisphere specialization. Moreover, the right hemisphere also seems to be well equipped for spatial processing. This neural substrate may result in the cognitive profile, at least in the majority of dyslexic boys (25), of intact and overused spatial, holistic processing combined with deficient linguistic, sequential processing. This pattern of cognitive skills may lead to an inefficient and limited strategy for the reading of phonetically coded orthographies.

The dyslexics were able to perform as well as the normal boys on the dichhaptic letters test in spite of their apparent use of different cognitive strategies. This test is similar to reading in that both necessarily involve both cognitive processes. The good performance of the dyslexics on the dichhaptic letters test suggests that it may be possible to design an approach to reading that elicits an optimum balance between linguistic processing (the phonetic approach) and spatial processing ("look-say" method) which may allow dyslexics to progress in reading. Such an approach, however, would be constrained by the requirements of reading English orthography and the cognitive capacities of dyslexics.

In view of the possible existence of right-hemisphere specialization for spatial processing in normal boys of at least 6 years of age (10), and in view of the extensive data indicating the presence of many aspects of hemisphere special-

ization at birth or in the first few years of life (26), the evidence for bi-hemisphere representation of spatial functions in dyslexics until at least age 14 supports a theory of a qualitative neural deficit rather than a neural maturational lag (27).

I have previously hypothesized that normal girls have bilateral representation of spatial functions (10), yet they exhibit no reading difficulty. This is not necessarily paradoxical. If the brain is a sex organ, then what may be satisfactory for one sex may not be for the other. Moreover, dyslexic boys, unlike normal girls, may have a deficient left hemisphere. Sexual dimorphism in neural organization (10) plus the relatively lower incidence of dyslexia in females than males (1, 12) suggest that the neural substrate of dyslexia in females may be different from that in males. There is some evidence to support this (28).

In the present work, I have made no direct study of cognitive deficits of dyslexia. I investigated neural factors in dyslexia and, on the basis of hypothesized neural correlates, predicted a cognitive profile of deficits and biases, which appears to be consistent with other research. Such neural hypotheses allow for further more specific predictions of cognitive deficits in dyslexia, which might not be considered without this neurological framework associated with a large body of knowledge of brain-behavior relationships (29).

It may now be possible to define and relabel the disorder of developmental dyslexia more precisely. The syndrome is not so much a specific deficit in reading (as many clinicians well know, since speech, spelling, fine motor coordination, among others are often also deficient) but, rather, a "specific *cognitive* deficit." Different subgroups may have different patterns of cognitive deficits and biases (30). If the reading of any orthography depends on the particular cognitive functions that are impaired in the individual, only then will the disorder become manifest with reading difficulty as part of the syndrome.

The Dyslexic Child Two Years Later[*,1,2]

Edna J. Hunter[3]

Hadley M. Lewis

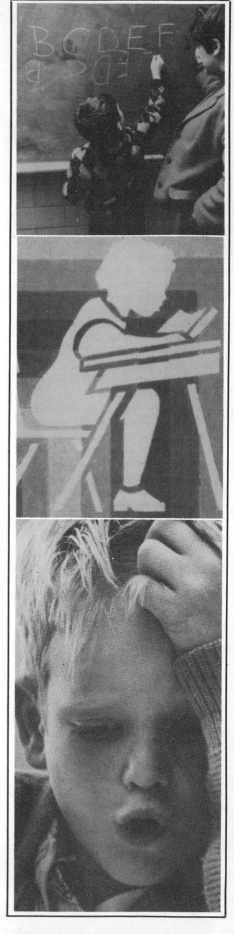

Summary

A follow-up was made of 18 male dyslexic children (RDs) and a group of matched controls (Cs), who had all been judged free from emotional and school adjustment problems two years earlier, (a) to see if RDs' reading deficit had been overcome, (b) to measure "emotional overlay," and (c) to find predictors of success in learning to read. Results showed that at the time of the follow-up (a) none of the RDs had overcome his reading disability despite remediational efforts; (b) RDs had significantly lower achievement levels and significantly more adjustment problems than Cs; (c) low scores for WISC Full Scale IQ, Vocabulary subtest, and Coding subtest were associated with large reading deficits two years later; and (d) high WISC Arithmetic and Coding subtest scores were associated with large gains in reading skill. Physiological measures did not predict size of deficit or gain in reading skill over time.

A. Introduction

The importance of early diagnosis of the potential dyslexic child to prevent permanent reading disability and to eliminate the emotional overlay which accumulates with repeated failure within the school environment has often been stressed. The present study was a two-year follow-up of 18 male non-readers, aged 9 years 6 months to 13 years 2 months, and a control group of average or above-average readers (matched by group) who had taken part in an earlier study (1, 2, 3). At the time of the initial study, parental and teacher reports and ratings showed that none of the children had appreciable emotional or behavioral adjustment problems within the home or school situation.

The purpose of the two-year follow-up was threefold: (a) to see if the large reading deficit of the nonreader had increased, decreased, or remained relatively stable over time; (b) to measure the "emotional overlay," if any, which had developed during the two-year interim; and (c) to discover which psychological, physiological, or developmental factors evident two years

* Received in the Editorial Office on November 27, 1972, and published immediately at Provincetown, Massachusetts. Copyright by The Journal Press.

[1] This research was accomplished at the U. S. Naval Hospital, San Diego, and was supported by Department of the Navy, Bureau of Medicine and Surgery, under Task No. MR006.02. The opinions and assertions contained herein are the private ones of the writers and are not to be construed as official or as reflecting the views of the Navy Department.

[2] The writers express their appreciation to Dr. Laverne C. Johnson for his helpful comments and to Ann Clay for typing the manuscript.

[3] Direct requests for reprints to the first author at the address shown at the end of this article.

earlier might have predicted which nonreaders would eventually overcome the reading disability and which ones would not.

B. Method

1. Subjects

Subjects were 18 of the 20 male reading disabled (RDs) children (e.g., children who demonstrated a one year or greater deficit in reading ability) who had taken part in the initial study and the 20 control (Cs) subjects of the previous study. At the time data were collected for the follow-up study, mean age for RDs was 11 years 7 months; for Cs, 11 years 8 months. Ages ranged from 9 years 6 months to 13 years 5 months ($N = 38$). Mean grade level for RDs was 6.1; for Cs, 6.5.

2. Procedure

Data obtained for each of the 38 children included scores on a recent test of reading skill (Wide Range Reading Test of the Wide Range Achievement Test) and teacher ratings of school behavior, academic achievement, and emotional adjustment. The Wechsler Intelligence Scale for Children (WISC) was not readministered for the follow-up; WISC scores from the earlier study were used for all analyses.

C. Results

1. Intellectual Levels

The RD and C groups were not significantly different for WISC Full Scale *IQ* (Full Scale $IQ = 115.3 \pm 10.2$, $N = 38$) or WISC Performance *IQ* (Performance $IQ = 111.4 \pm 10.5$, $N = 38$). The two groups differed significantly, however, on WISC Verbal *IQ* (two-tailed t test for independent means, $p < .001$). Mean Verbal *IQ* for RDs was 110.0 ± 10.4; for Cs, 122.5 ± 10.3.

2. Achievement Levels

On the basis of teacher ratings, there were statistically significant differences between the groups at the time of the follow-up with respect to achievement in all school subjects, as shown in Figure 1. These differences reached the .01 level of significance for mathematics and social studies, and the .001 level for reading and language achievement (two-tailed t tests for uncorrelated means).

3. Reading Skills—Two Years Later

Of the 18 RD children in the follow-up, all but one child had received remedial assistance in language skills of some kind during the two-year interim; e.g., special classes in remedial reading, classes for the educationally handicapped, individual instruction, etc. In spite of remedial efforts, *not one of the 18 children had overcome his reading disability.* All RDs continued to demonstrate reading deficits equal to one year or more below expected age-grade reading level. Two years earlier, mean reading deficit for RDs was 2.5 years; data from the follow-up showed a mean deficit of 2.9 years, with deficits ranging from 1.0 years to as high as 5.5 years.

Data from the original study had shown statistically significant differences between readers and nonreaders for scores on the Bender Visual Gestalt Test; the WISC Verbal *IQ;* the WISC Information, Arithmetic, Similarities, Vocabulary, Digit Span, Picture Completion, and Coding subtests; tested laterality; familial incidence of dyslexia; birthdate in relation to school year; motor reaction time; skin conductance level; number electrodermal offset responses; and heart rate variability. Full reports of

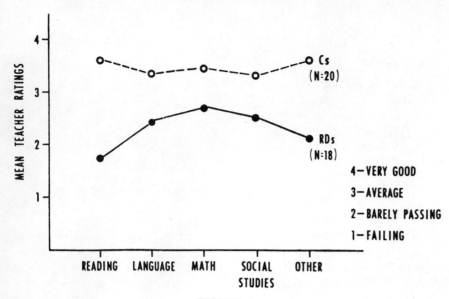

ACHIEVEMENT LEVEL

4—VERY GOOD
3—AVERAGE
2—BARELY PASSING
1—FAILING

FIGURE 1

DIFFERENCES IN MEAN ACHIEVEMENT LEVELS IN SCHOOL SUBJECTS FOR NONREADERS (RDs)
AND MATCHED CONTROLS (Cs) BASED UPON TEACHER RATINGS

these findings appear elsewhere (1, 2, 3).

For nonreaders, correlation coefficients between absolute gains in reading skills made in the two-year period and measures taken two years previously showed that the only measures with predictive validity were the WISC Arithmetic subtest score and the WISC Coding subtest score (see Table 1). Subjects with higher scores showed the greatest reading gains. Those RDs

TABLE 1

CORRELATIONS BETWEEN PSYCHOPHYSIOLOGICAL MEASURES FOR NONREADERS TAKEN TWO
YEARS PREVIOUSLY AND GAIN IN READING SKILL AND MAGNITUDE
OF READING DEFICIT TWO YEARS LATER

Measure	Reading gain	Reading deficit
Test measures		
Bender Gestalt Visual Motor Test	.06	.15
WISC Full Scale *IQ*	—.19	—.45*
WISC subtests		
Information	—.16	—.31
Vocabulary	.35	—.58**
Arithmetic	.60**	—.36
Similarities	—.30	.02
Digit Span	—.04	—.07
Picture Completion	.13	—.08
Coding	.54**	—.65**
Physiological measures		
Motor reaction time	—.08	.35
Electrodermal response (number offset responses)	—.02	.15
Skin conductance level (decrease over time)	—.22	.32
Heart rate variability (standard deviation of the beat-by-beat heart rate)	.28	.26

Note: N = 18.
* *p* < .05.
** *p* < .01.

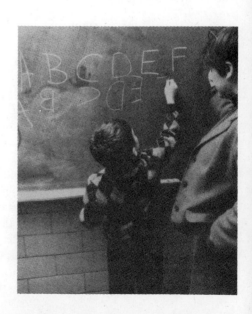

with the highest WISC Full Scale *IQ* scores did not necessarily make the largest gains in reading skill over time. However, subjects with lower Full Scale WISC *IQ*s at fourth grade level had larger reading deficits present at sixth grade level ($r = -.45$, $p < .05$, $N = 18$). Larger reading deficits were also associated with lower scores on the WISC Vocabulary subtest ($r = -.58$, $p < .01$, $N = 18$) and on the WISC Coding subtest ($r = -.65$, $p < .01$, $N = 18$). None of the physiological measures taken at the time of the earlier study correlated significantly with magnitude of the reading deficit two years later.

At the time of the initial study the younger half of the RD group did not differ from the older half with respect to magnitude of the reading deficit. Mean deficit for younger RDs was 2.7 years, as compared with a deficit of 2.3 years for the older RDs. However, two years later, mean reading deficit for the younger half was 3.8 years; for the older RDs, 2.0 years. This difference between the younger and older nonreaders was statistically significant at the .001 level (two-tailed *t* test for uncorrelated means).

As expected, Cs were still significantly better readers than RDs two years after the initial study (two-tailed *t* test for independent means, $p < .001$). At the time of the follow-up, Cs showed a mean reading acceleration above expected age-grade level of 1.7 years. Acceleration shown two years earlier was 1.9 years. Reading levels for the majority of Cs were approximately equal to those demonstrated two years previously, although one control subject (Full Scale WISC *IQ* = 112) would now be categorized as "reading disabled"; that is, he was at least one year below expected age-grade level. Three control subjects were even more highly accelerated than two years previously; two tested more than five years above expected age-grade level in reading skill. (Mean Full Scale WISC *IQ* for those two Ss was 130.0, which was considerably higher than the mean for the group as a whole.)

4. *Did an Emotional Overlay Develop over Time?*

For the original study, only those children were included who showed no apparent emotional problems and were not behavioral problems within the school situation on the basis of parental and teacher reports and personal interviews. Data from the first study showed only two "adjustment" measures on which RDs differed significantly from the control group. The RDs were rated as less self-confident than Cs by their mothers and were rated by the experimenter as displaying more hyperactivity during the laboratory session.

Two years later, however, there were a large number of differences between the two groups with respect to emotional and school adjustment problems (see Figure 2). On the basis of scores from a teacher rating scale, there were highly significant differences between RDs and Cs with respect to the ability to concentrate, oversensitivity, temper outbursts, and stubbornness (two-tailed *t* test for independent means, $p < .01$). The RD child was also judged significantly more excitable, selfish, quarrelsome, defiant, and attention-demanding. He "tattled" more, tended to be a greater disturbance to other children, and was more apt to "fall apart" under stress (two-tailed *t* test for independent means, $p < .05$).

D. DISCUSSION

The present study was a two-year follow-up of 18 reading disabled male children, aged 9 years 6 months to 13 years 2 months, and a matched control group. Scores on the Wide Range Reading Test, school achievement scores in related subjects, and behavioral ratings by teachers showed that during the two-year interval, in no instance was the nonreader's deficit overcome, and an "emotional overlay" was apparent for the RDs which was not present for the controls. The teacher rating scale used for the follow-up was not identical with that used for the initial study. Therefore, it is possible that

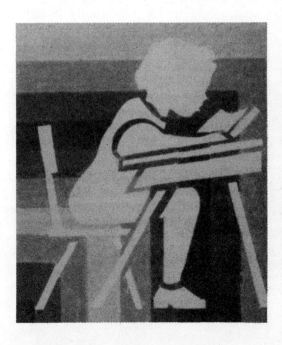

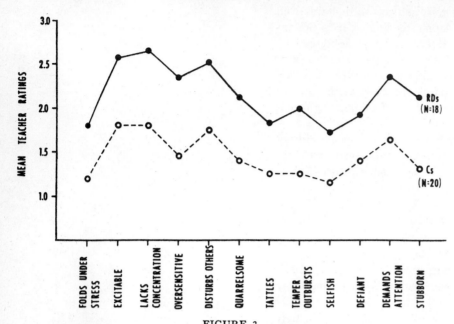

CLASSROOM BEHAVIOR

FIGURE 2
THE DEGREE TO WHICH VARIOUS CLASSROOM BEHAVIORS WERE DISPLAYED BY
NONREADERS (RDs) AND A MATCHED CONTROL GROUP (Cs)
BASED UPON TEACHER RATINGS
Ratings were as follows: 4 = Excessive; 3 = Often; 2 = Occasionally; and 1 = Never.
All between-group differences were statistically significant at the .05 level or better.

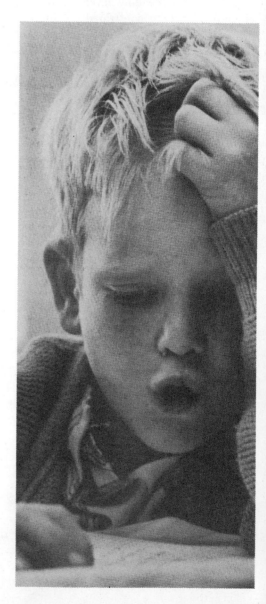

these adjustment and emotional differences between the groups were present to some extent two years earlier.

Correlation coefficients between magnitude of the reading deficit at the time of the follow-up study and measures taken two years earlier indicate that low scores on the WISC Full Scale *IQ*, the WISC Vocabulary subtest, and the WISC Coding subtest were significantly related to large reading deficits two years later. The WISC Arithmetic subtest score and Coding sub-test score were significantly and positively related to increases in reading ability over time (WISC Arithmetic, $r = +.60$; WISC Coding, $r = +.54$; $p < .01$). None of the physiological measures (motor reaction time, skin conductance level, electrodermal offset response, heart rate variability) was found to be related significantly to future reading deficit or to increase in reading skill over the two-year period.

The mean reading deficit of the older half of the RD group was approximately equal in magnitude to the mean for that half found at the time of the initial study. The younger half of the RD group showed a significantly larger mean deficit than was evident previously. In the selection of subjects for the initial study, children were considered as reading disabled if demonstrated reading skills fell at least one full year or more below expected age-grade level. It may be that the earlier a reading deficit is recognized, the more serious the deficit. In other words, a one-year deficit at third grade level is a greater deficit than a one-year deficit at fifth grade level.

In a recent study, Maginnis (4) found that those children with the largest reading deficits are not necessarily the ones who will profit most from re-mediation. Data from this follow-up study showed a negligible correlation ($r = +.05$, $N = 18$) between the degree of reading disability present two years earlier and the size of gain in reading skills after two years. Retrospectively, the correlations between reading deficit at time of follow-up and the gain in skill over the preceding two years was $-.60$ ($p < .01$, $N = 18$). Not one of the dyslexic children had overcome his reading disability, and nearly half the group ($N = 8$) made only minimal progress—in spite of special remediational procedures. In many cases, the child who was reading at second grade level when he was in the fourth grade was still reading at approximately the second grade level when he was in the sixth grade. It is not surprising that serious emotional and school adjustment problems appeared to develop over the two-year period.

Silberberg and Silberberg (5) have pointed to seven recent studies which indicate that children subjected to remedial reading show only small short-term positive effects. Those authors emphasized that reading is but a "tool" to educate, and when it becomes evident that a child is unable to learn to read, perhaps another educative tool should be considered. Results of the present study show that the "emotional cost" of not learning to read is exceedingly high for the dyslexic child, and the "return" on remedial investment exceedingly low. We need another tool!

REFERENCES

1. HUNTER, E. J. Autonomic responses to aircraft noise in dyslexic children. *Psychol. in Sch.,* 1971, **8**, 362-367.
2. HUNTER, E. J., & JOHNSON, L. C. Developmental and psychological differences between readers and nonreaders. *J. Learn. Disabil.,* 1971, **4**, 572-577.
3. HUNTER, E. J., JOHNSON, L. C., & KEEFE, F. B. Electrodermal and cardiovascular responses in nonreaders. *J. Learn. Disabil.,* 1972, **5**, 187-197.
4. MAGINNIS, G. H. Reading disability and remedial gain. *J. Learn. Disabil.,* 1971, **4**, 322-324.
5. SILBERBERG, N. E., & SILBERBERG, M. C. The bookless curriculum: An educational alternative. *J. Learn. Disabil.,* 1969, **2**, 302-307.

Navy Medical Neuropsychiatric Research Unit
San Diego, California 92152

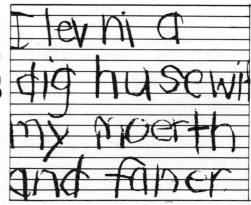

Reading Disability:
An Information-Processing Analysis

Abstract. *In a task designed to separate perceptual processes from memory, 12-year-old children with reading disabilities showed no perceptual deficits as compared to their peers. However, they exhibited major deficiencies in memory skills for both labelable and nonlabelable visual information. Reading-disabled children in this age group appear to suffer from a basic information-processing deficiency.*

FREDERICK J. MORRISON
BRUNO GIORDANI, JILL NAGY

The nature of reading disability has been one of the most difficult and puzzling problems facing psychologists and educators. For years reading problems were thought to be a difficulty in the perception of written symbols. As recently as 1972 Cruickshank concluded that reading disabilities "... are essentially and almost always the result of perceptual problems based on the neurological system" (*1*). However, recent work has cast doubt on this "perceptual deficit" hypothesis and pointed instead to deficits in memory processes (*2*). One persistent problem in assessing reading disability has been the inability to devise experimental procedures for separating perception from memory (*3*). Recently techniques have been developed for isolating perceptual and memory processes by assuming them to be occurring sequentially in time (*4*). It has been demonstrated experimentally that initially large amounts of information are perceived by the visual system. This information persists in a raw perceptual form (called visual information storage or VIS) for about 0.25 second. During this period subjects are actively coding and transferring information into a more permanent storage (called short-term storage). The ability to temporally separate perception from memory in the present study made possible a more fine-grained assessment of some factors potentially underlying reading disability. The specific procedure used was called the partial report technique. It involved presenting subjects with a circular array of eight visual forms for a very brief duration (150 msec) which prevented eye movements. Following offset of the array at varying intervals (0 to 2000 msec) a teardrop indicator appeared under one of the forms. The subject's task was to report the form to which the indicator had pointed by picking it out on a response card that

contained all eight of the forms used in the original array. By noting the accuracy levels at the various delay intervals it was possible to estimate the amount of information initially perceived by the subject (0-msec delay), the trace duration of information in VIS (0 to 300 msec), and the amount of information encoded and transferred to more permanent storage (300 to 2000 msec). It was hypothesized that if reading disability were a perceptual deficit, then performance of reading-disabled children would be inferior to that of normal readers at short delays (0 to 300 msec) for which information was still held in a raw perceptual form. However, if reading disability involved an encoding or memory deficit, it was believed that performance of poor readers would be inferior only at later intervals (after the 300-msec delay). Also included in this study was a test of whether reading disability was a specific deficit, limited to primarily verbal materials (letters), or whether it might be a more general processing deficit. Accordingly three sets of figures that had been shown to differ in degree of familiarity or labelability were used (*5*): letters, geometric forms, and abstract forms (Fig. 1). It was thought that if reading disability were limited to predominantly verbal materials, major differences in performance between normal and poor readers would occur only with the letter stimuli or possibly geometric forms. If, however, reading-disabled children suffered a more general processing deficit, major differences were expected on all three sets of forms.

The children tested were all 12-year-old males in the sixth grade. Two groups of nine children each were identified as either normal readers (reading at grade level) or poor readers (reading at two levels or more below grade level) on the Comprehensive Test of Basic Skills

(McGraw-Hill). The poor readers were average or above in intelligence and in other school subjects, and showed no gross behavioral problems or organic disorders. The poor readers were all in regular classes and had not received special instruction. A Gerbrands four-field tachistoscope, coupled with six Hunter timers which controlled stimulus durations and other intervals, was used in the experiment. After being familiarized with the equipment and procedure, each subject went through the following sequence: he looked inside the tachistoscope at a small fixation dot in the center of the visual field; a "ready-go" signal was given verbally and, after a 750-msec delay, the stimulus array flashed on for 150 msec. Following offset of the array the indicator appeared under one of the figures for 50 msec followed by reappearance of the fixation field. The subject then chose the indicated figure on the response card. Each stimulus card contained eight forms (each subtending 33′ of visual angle) in a circular array 1.30° in radius from central fixation. The teardrop indicator, subtending 26′ of visual angle, was placed approximately 25′ of visual angle from the stimulus figure. Illumination levels for the stimulus field, indicator field, and fixation field were approximately 4.0 foot-lamberts. Ten delay intervals were sampled: 0, 50, 100, 200, 300, 500, 800, 1000, 1500, and 2000 msec. A total of eight cards per delay interval was presented. Each position in the array served once as target position and each stimulus served as target stimulus once per interstimulus interval. All subjects were tested on the three familiarity sets on three consecutive days. For half the subjects the order of presentation was letters, geometric forms, and abstract forms while the other half viewed abstract forms followed by geometric forms and letters. A total of 80 trials per

"Reading Disability: An Information-Processing Analysis," *Science*, Vol. 196 No. 4285, April 1, 1977. ©1977 The American Association for the Advancement of Science.

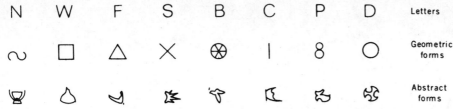

Fig. 1. Complete set of letters, geometric forms, and abstract forms used in the stimulus arrays.

familiarity set was presented.

The mean number of correct responses made by the normal and poor readers was compared across two sets of delay intervals: the perceptual phase, 0 to 300 msec and the encoding-memory phase, 500 to 2000 msec. Four major findings stood out. (i) There was no difference in performance between normal and poor readers across the 0- to 300-msec delay interval. As shown in Fig. 2, poor readers performed as well as normal readers while the information was present perceptually. (ii) No differences were found between the two groups during this phase on any of the sets of visual forms. (iii) Normal readers performed significantly better than poor readers during the encoding-memory phase ($P <$ .0001). (iv) This superiority held for all three sets of forms (6).

Although it was clear from the first two results that the quantity of information initially perceived by poor readers was identical to that of normal readers, the quality of information might have been different in the two groups. At short delay intervals the poor readers might still have had enough high-quality information to perform adequately but at later intervals when information was fading rapidly the lower quality of information perceived by the poor readers could have produced lower levels of perform-

ance. In order to test this possibility a stimulus-response confusion matrix was constructed for each reading group and set of forms separately for each of the two sets of delay intervals. On the basis of these group matrices, a configuration of items representing their judged similarity was determined by a multi-dimensional scaling analysis (7). It was thought that by observing the kinds of

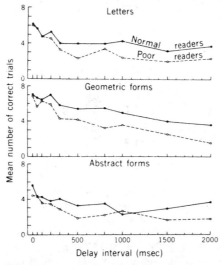

Fig. 2. Accuracy levels of normal and poor readers on the three sets of figures across all delay intervals.

confusions made by the two groups of readers, an assessment could be made of whether they differed in the kind or qual-

ity of information perceived. Across all sets of figures and delay intervals, normal and poor readers showed similar confusion error patterns. Both groups tended to choose an incorrect form that was visually confusable with the correct form.

Taken together, the results of this study showed that poor readers were not deficient in the quantity or quality of information they initially perceived or in the trace duration of that information in a raw perceptual form (VIS). Poor readers did show a striking deficit during the 300- to 2000-msec interval, which argues that reading disability involves some problem in the processing of information in stages following initial perception, perhaps in encoding, organizational, or retrieval skills. Also, reading disability is not limited to verbal materials since poor readers performed equally poorly compared with normal readers on the geometric and abstract forms. The real difficulty may involve a more abstract ability which underlies processing of both labelable and unlabelable forms. The conclusions drawn from this study must at present be restricted to older children since beginning readers were not included. Further research is needed to assess the generality across age of the processing deficit discovered here. Nevertheless, the fact that poor readers were found to be deficient in a form of processing that is not primarily verbal is important especially given a recent tendency to tie reading problems in older children to verbal and linguistic processes (4). The development of techniques that can tease apart component processes acting on information represents an important step toward clarifying the complex nature of reading disability.

Dyslexia: A hemispheric explanation

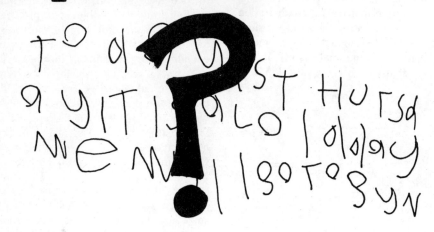

Handwriting of Mike: 10 years old

Learning to read English is not especially difficult. Most children master the task within six or seven years of age. But when d's look like b's and when p's look like q's, the job of learning to read becomes a serious challenge. Confusion in the spatial orientation of letters is among the problems faced by children who suffer from a clinical syndrome known as developmental dyslexia. The disorder affects as many as 5 percent of school-aged children in the United States who are otherwise intellectually, emotionally and medically normal. Even though such children may have no other serious problem, the difficulty in learning their letters is particularly incapacitating in modern, highly literate societies and frequently results in serious secondary behavioral and emotional problems.

Dyslexia and its effects have been recognized for years, but plausible explanations of its cause have been hard to come by. Neurological, social and educational factors have been implicated, but none has received strong or consistent support—until now. One long-standing hypothesis, originally suggested in 1937, implicates abnormal cerebral dominance or functional asymmetry of the brain's hemispheres. With the recent explosion of research on left-right hemisphere processes, it has become possible to test this hypothesis. In the Jan. 21 SCIENCE Sandra F. Witelson of McMaster University in Ha-milton, Ontario, reports that dyslexia may be associated with representation of spatial data (including alphabet letters) in both hemispheres, instead of primarily in the right as is the usual case.

Witelson's findings are based on studies of 85 right-handed boys, 6 to 14 years of age (the condition is seen most often in males), who were administered a battery of tests commonly used to determine hemispheric specialization. The results were compared with those of 156 control subjects. Evidence for bilateral representation of spatial functions was found among the dyslexic children. Dual representation of a cognitive process such as spatial perception could, says Witelson, "affect cognition by overloading one hemisphere [the left, in this case] and interfering with those functions 'native' to it." The functions native to the left hemisphere include sequential and linguistic processing. Interference with such processes would lead to poor performance in linguistic tasks and reading.

The fact that spatial processing appears to be represented in both hemispheres in dyslexic children suggests, says Witelson, "that it may be possible to design an approach to reading that elicits an optimum balance between linguistic processing (the phonetic approach and spatial processing ("look-say" method) which may allow dyslexics to progress in reading."

Handwriting of Allen: 10 years old

"Dyslexia: A Hemispheric Explanation," *Science News*, Vol. 111 No. 4, January 22, 1977. ®1977 Science Service, Inc.

COMMONLY REVERSED WORDS:

WAS
STEP
SAW
TAP
PAN
COP

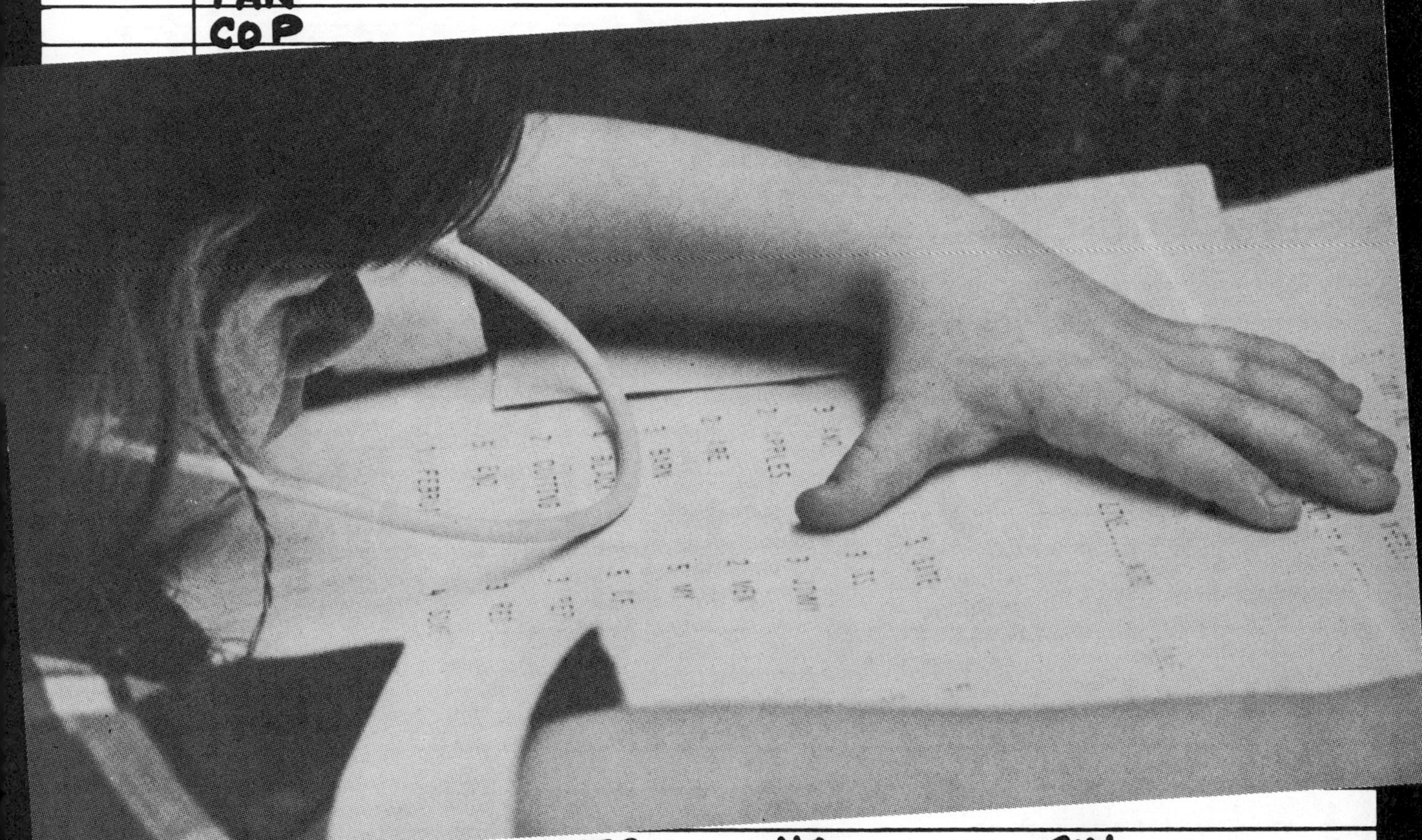

PAL	RATS	NO	PIN
ON	NIP	SPOT	TUB
TIP	LAP	NET	TRAP
POT	STAR	PART	RAT
NAP	PIT	TOPS	TEN
TAR	PETS	PAT	BUT

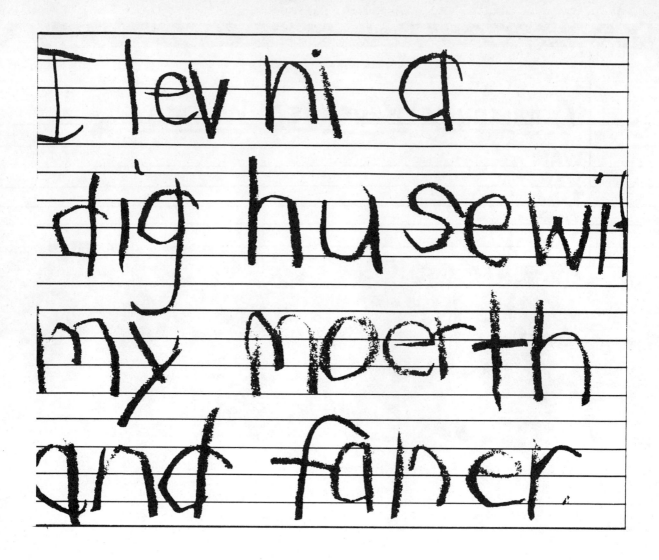

I lev ni a
dig husewif
my moerth
and faner

STAFF

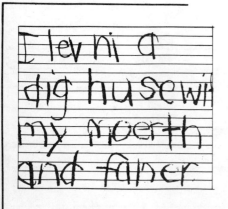

Publisher	John Quirk
Editor	Joseph Logan
Editor	Rodney Mulock
Director of Design	Donald Burns
Photographer	Richard Pawlikowski
Program Coordinator	Susan Allen
Staff Consultant	Dona Chiappe
Editorial Assistant	Helen Flynn

Cover Design

Li Bailey of Enoch and Eisenman Inc. New York City.

Appendix: Agencies and Services for Exceptional Children

Alexander Graham Bell Association for the Deaf, Inc.
Volta Bureau for the Deaf
3417 Volta Place, NW
Washington, D.C. 20007

American Academy of Pediatrics
1801 Hinman Avenue
Evanston, Illinois 60204

American Association for Gifted Children
15 Gramercy Park
New York, N.Y. 10003

American Association on Mental Deficiency
5201 Connecticut Avenue, NW
Washington, D.C. 20015

American Association of Psychiatric Clinics for
Children
250 West 57th Street
New York, N.Y.

American Bar Association
Commission on the Mentally Disabled
1800 M Street, NW
Washington, D.C. 20036

American Foundation for the Blind
15 W. 16th Street
New York, N.Y. 10011

American Medical Association
535 N. Dearborn Street
Chicago, Illinois 60610

American Speech and Hearing Association
9030 Old Georgetown Road
Washington, D.C. 20014

Association for the Aid of Crippled Children
345 E. 46th Street
New York, N.Y. 10017

Association for Children with Learning Disabilities
2200 Brownsville Road
Pittsburgh, Pennsylvania 15210

Association for Education of the Visually
Handicapped
1604 Spruce Street
Philadelphia, Pennsylvania 19103

Association for the Help of Retarded Children
200 Park Avenue, South
New York, N.Y.

Association for the Visually Handicapped
1839 Frankfort Avenue
Louisville, Kentucky 40206

Center on Human Policy
Division of Special Education and Rehabilitation
Syracuse University
Syracuse, New York 13210

Child Fund
275 Windsor Street
Hartford, Connecticut 06120

Children's Defense Fund
520 New Hampshire Avenue NW
Washington, D.C. 20036

Closer Look
National Information Center for the Handicapped
1201 Sixteenth Street NW
Washington, D.C. 20036

Clifford W. Beers Guidance Clinic
432 Temple Street
New Haven, Connecticut 06510

Child Study Center
Yale University
333 Cedar Street
New Haven, Connecticut 06520

Child Welfare League of America, Inc.
44 East 23rd Street
New York, N.Y. 10010

Children's Bureau
United States Department of Health, Education
and Welfare
Washington, D.C.

Council for Exceptional Children
1411 Jefferson Davis Highway
Arlington, Virginia 22202

Epilepsy Foundation of America
1828 "L" Street NW
Washington, D.C. 20036

Gifted Child Society, Inc.
59 Glen Gray Road
Oakland, New Jersey 07436

Institute for the Study of Mental Retardation
and Related Disabilities
130 South First
University of Michigan
Ann Arbor, Michigan 48108

International Association for the Scientific Study
of Mental Deficiency
Ellen Horn, AAMD
5201 Connecticut Avenue NW
Washington, D.C. 20015

International League of Societies for the Mentally
Handicapped
Rue Forestiere 12
Brussels, Belgium

Joseph P. Kennedy, Jr. Foundation
1701 K Street NW
Washington, D.C. 20006

League for Emotioally Disturbed Children
171 Madison Avenue
New York, N.Y.

Muscular Dystrophy Associations of America
1790 Broadway
New York, N.Y. 10019

National Aid to the Visually Handicapped
3201 Balboa Street
San Francisco, California 94121

National Association of Coordinators of State
Programs for the Mentally Retarded
2001 Jefferson Davis Highway
Arlington, Virginai 22202

National Association of Hearing and Speech
Agencies
919 18th Street NW
Washington, D.C. 20006

National Association for Creative Children and
Adults
8080 Springvalley Drive
Cincinnati, Ohio 45236
(Mrs. Ann F. Isaacs, Executive Director)

National Association for Retarded Children
420 Lexington Avenue
New York, N.Y.

National Association for Retarded Citizens
2709 Avenue E East
Arlington, Texas 76010

National Children's Rehabilitation Center
P.O. Box 1260
Leesburg, Virginia

National Association for the Visually Handicapped
3201 Balboa Street
San Francisco, California 94121

National Association of the Deaf
814 Thayer Avenue
Silver Spring, Maryland 20910

National Cystic Fibrosis Foundation
3379 Peachtree Road NE
Atlanta, Georgia 30326

National Easter Seal Society for Crippled Children
and Adults
2023 W. Ogden Avenue
Chicago, Illinois 60612

National Federation of the Blind
218 Randolph Hotel
Des Moines, Iowa 50309

National Paraplegia Foundation
333 N. Michigan Avenue
Chicago, Illinois 60601

National Society for Autistic Children
621 Central Avenue
Albany, N.Y. 12206

National Society for Prevention of Blindness, Inc.
79 Madison Avenue
New York, N.Y. 10016

Orton Society, Inc.
8415 Bellona Lane
Baltimore, Maryland 21204

President's Committee on Mental Retardation
Regional Office Building #3
7th and D Streets SW
Room 2614
Washington, D.C. 20201

United Cerebral Palsy Associations
66 E 34th Street
New York, N.Y. 10016

Special Learning Corporation's
For: Mainstreaming, Special Education Teachers

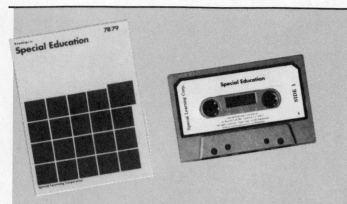

SPECIAL EDUCATION

This seminar provides an overview of special education.
1. Special Education: An Historical Perspective
2. Methodology
3. Mental Retardaton
4. Emotional and Behavioral Disorders
5. Physically and Sensorially Handicapped
6. Learning Disabilites
7. Psychology of Exceptional Children

$24.50

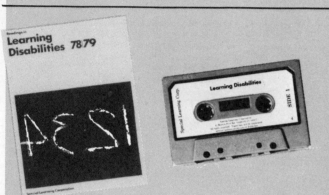

LEARNING DISABILITIES

Discussion of learning disabilities and physical neurological approach to education.
1. Dimensions of Learning Disabilities
2. Diagnosis and Assessment
3. Perceptual Disorders
4. Motor Activity Disorders
5. Language Disorders
6. Reading Disorders
7. Social Emotional Problems of the Learning Disabled

$24.50

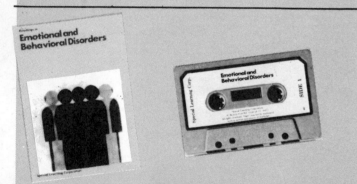

EMOTIONAL AND BEHAVIOR DISORDERS

Understanding the difficult child.
1. Emotional Disorders:
    A Perspective
2. Emotional and Behavioral Disorders in the Classroom
3. Hyperkinesis
4. Deviant Behavior and Juvenile Delinquency
5. Behavior Therapies

$24.50

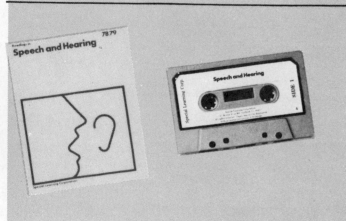

SPEECH AND HEARING

The remarkable ability of brain, tongue and ear in use of speech.
1. Physiological Auditory Impairment: Diagnosis and Assessment
2. Speech Disorders: Pathology and Classification
3. Linguistic Development
4. Cognitive and Communicative Skills
5. Educational Services: Resources and Therapies
6. Research and Rehabilitation: Medical, Technological and Psychological

$24.50

Teacher-Training Series

Administrators, PL 94-142, Special Schools

VISUALLY HANDICAPPED EDUCATION

A discussion of 4 phases in blind and visually handicapped education.

1. Education of the Visually Handicapped: Historical Overview
2. Etiology of Visual Impairment: Research
3. Cognitive and Communicative Skills
4. Perceptual Disorders
5. Vocational and Educational Support Systems
6. Socialization and Rehabilitation

$24.50

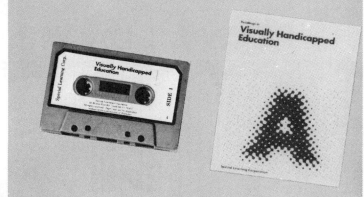

AUTISM

Hostile attitudes, interpersonal relationships with emphasis on clinical problems.

1. Concept of Autism: History and Theory
2. Prospectus on Causes
3. Development of Perceptual Skills
4. Behavioral Therapy
5. Language Development

$24.50

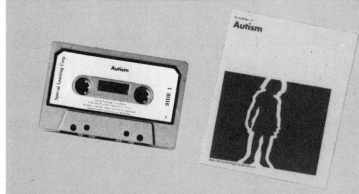

GIFTED AND TALENTED EDUCATION

The subject of identification, leadership, creativity, guidance and educating promising youth.

1. Perspective on Gifted Education: Identification
2. Programming for the Academically Talented
3. Curriculum and Materials....Methodology
4. Placement: Mainstreaming vs. Special Programming
5. Community Resources and Support Services

$43.50

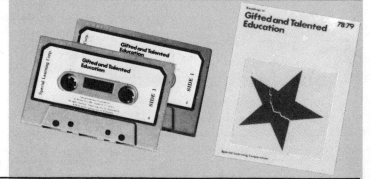

DIAGNOSIS AND PLACEMENT

1. Current Testing Procedures
2. Personality Assessment
3. Cognitive Assessment
4. Medical Assessment
5. Placement: Self-Contained or Mainstreamed

Individual intelligence testing is discussed as well as identification of children in need of special help and of gifted, mentally retarded and emotionally disturbed.

$43.50

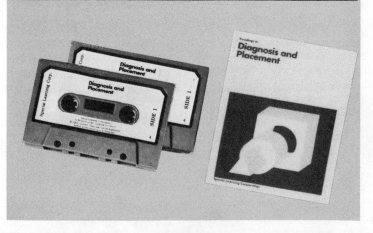

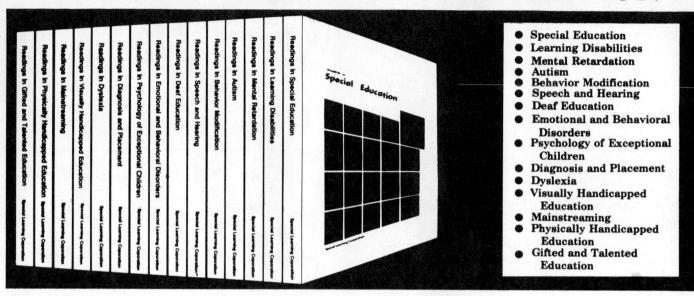

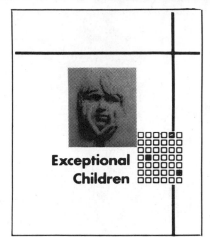

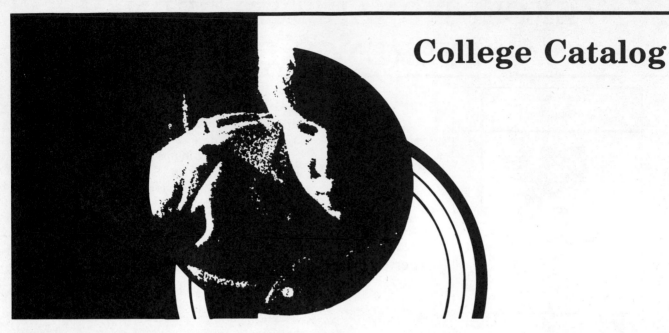

CUSTOM PUBLISHING

CUSTOM-PUBLISHED BOOKS
FOR YOUR COURSE OF STUDY

TEXTS DESIGNED FOR YOUR COURSE

Special Learning Corporation publishes books that are particularly tailored for a specific course and that fit a professor's specific needs. Special Learning Corporation will compile a book of required readings based on a bibliography selected by the professor teaching the course. These selected academic readings serve as the required course of readings and in some cases the major book for the course. It also benefits other small enrollment areas at various other colleges. Originally designed to serve small course areas in special education, e.g. *Readings for Teachers of Minimally Brain Damaged Children*, the idea spread to larger course enrollments in Special Education, Psychology, and Education.

HOW DOES CUSTOM PUBLISHING WORK?

- A professor selects a list of articles relevant to his course from a bibliography. These articles usually come from scholarly journals, magazines. The professor can also suggest other articles, unpublished papers, and articles he has written.
- Special Learning Corporation does all editoral work, clears permissions and produces the book--using the facsimile reproduction of the articles.
- The book is then used in the professor's course of study.

Pages: 192 to 224 or about 50 to 70 articles.
Price: $5.95 to $6.95 (Hardback available to libraries for $12.00).

For more information please contact:

Custom Publishing Division,
Special Learning Corporation

Special Learning Corporation
42 Boston Post Rd. Guilford, Connecticut 06437

1978 Catalog
SPECIAL LEARNING CORPORATION

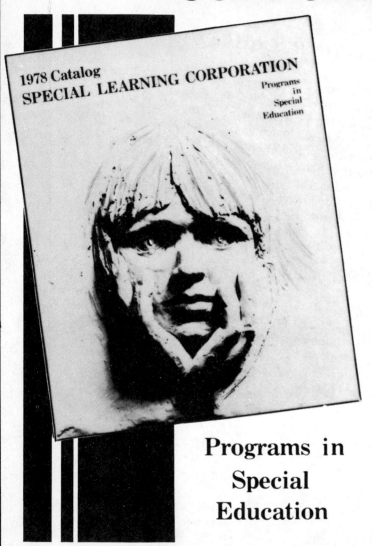

1978 Catalog
SPECIAL LEARNING CORPORATION
Programs in Special Education

Programs in Special Education

- special education ● learning disabilities ● mental retardation
- autism ● behavior modification ● mainstreaming ● gifted and talented
- physically handicapped ● deaf education ● speech and hearing
- emotional and behavioral disorders ● visually handicapped
- diagnosis and placement ● psychology of exceptional children

Special Learning Corporation
42 Boston Post Rd. Guilford, Connecticut 06437 (203) 453-6212

COMMENTS PLEASE:

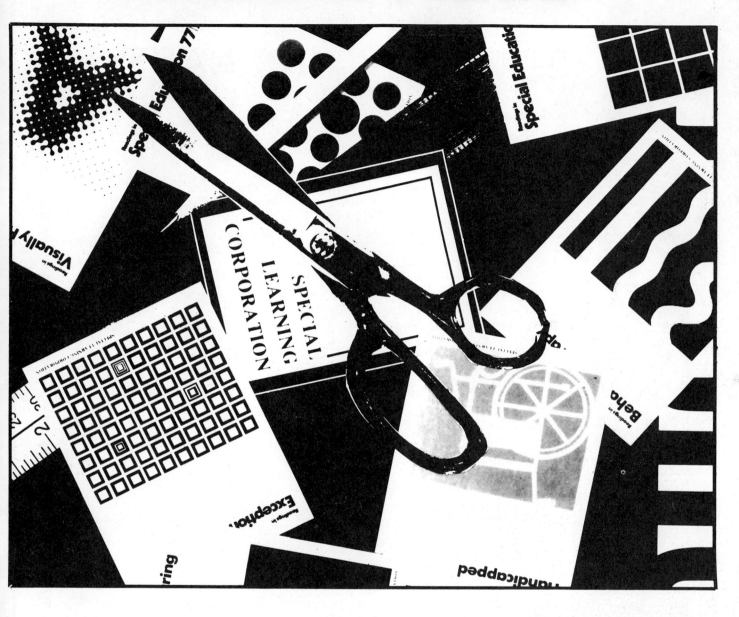

SPECIAL LEARNING CORPORATION

42 Boston Post Rd.

Guilford, Conn. 06437

SPECIAL LEARNING CORPORATION

COMMENTS PLEASE:

Does this book fit your course of study?

Why? (Why not?)

Is this book useable for other courses of study? Please list.

What other areas would you like us to publish in using this format?

What type of exceptional child are you interested in learning more about?

Would you use this as a basic text?

How many students are enrolled in these course areas?

_____ Special Education _____ Mental Retardation _____ Psychology _____ Emotional Disorders

_____ Exceptional Children _____ Learning Disabilities   Other _____

Do you want to be sent a copy of our elementary student materials catalog?

Do you want a copy of our college catalog?

Would you like a copy of our next edition? ☐ yes ☐ no

Are you a ☐ student or an ☐ instructor?

Your name _____ school _____

Term used _____ Date _____

address _____

city _____ state _____ zip _____

telephone number _____

D